9 Essentials for Quality Health Outcomes in Older and High-Risk Patients

Health care systems today face an impending crisis. An increasingly aging population with high-risk patients and rising costs challenges most teams in providing meaningful, lasting patient outcomes. This book provides a fresh perspective, shifting focus from rigid clinical protocols to humanistic elements of patient care, emphasizing empathy, communication, and rapport-building. It offers tangible interprofessional team-based solutions for immediate actionable results through case studies, interactive exercises, and real-life patient scenarios while also tackling burn-out, disengagement, and team communication. Blending humor, inspiration, and practical insights, complex health care challenges become more relatable and engaging for clinicians and health care administrators.

Key Features:

- *Concrete strategies for managing complex patients*: Offers a blueprint for patient success in various challenging situations. Equips readers with specific, actionable strategies that can be directly applied to their practice, helping them overcome the paralysis that often accompanies complex patient care.
- *Case-based complex patient examples*: Provides readers with practical, real-life scenarios for understanding and navigating the intricacies of managing complex patients. This hands-on approach helps bridge the gap between

theory and practice, making the information more relatable and actionable. Readers learn not just theoretical concepts but also how to implement effective solutions in real-world situations.

- *Interactive reflections reinforcing learning concepts*: End-of-chapter reflections inspire critical thinking with deeper understanding while reinforcing key ideas helping readers apply concepts to their own practice.
- *Engaging reading*: Keeps readers invested and motivated through a mix of humor, inspiration, and storytelling. The immigrant family's narrative of struggle with complex care developed with each key concept throughout the book humanizes principles in a compelling way, making them more memorable and impactful.

9 Essentials for Quality Health Outcomes in Older and High-Risk Patients
An Interprofessional Handbook

Robert S. Vaidya

CRC Press
Taylor & Francis Group
Boca Raton London New York

CRC Press is an imprint of the
Taylor & Francis Group, an **informa** business

Designed cover image: IStock

First edition published 2026
by CRC Press
2385 NW Executive Center Drive, Suite 320, Boca Raton FL 33431

and by CRC Press
4 Park Square, Milton Park, Abingdon, Oxon, OX14 4RN

CRC Press is an imprint of Taylor & Francis Group, LLC

ISBN: 978-1-041-10451-3 (hbk)
ISBN: 978-1-041-10450-6 (pbk)
ISBN: 978-1-003-65508-4 (ebk)

DOI: 10.1201/9781003655084

Typeset in Sabon
by SPi Technologies India Pvt Ltd (Straive)

To my wife, Carolyn. Without you,
none of this was possible.

To my daughters, Audrey and Cailyn.
I love you more than words can say.

To Mom and Dad, your guidance, support, and undying belief in
me allowed me to reach great heights and fulfil my dreams.

Contents

About the Author

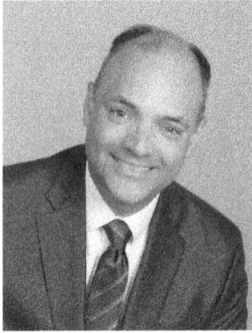

Robert S. Vaidya is a practicing board-certified internal medicine physician with BA in Psychology and a master's degree in public health. Dr. Vaidya has extensive experience in high-risk value-based health care, including the Henry Ford Medical Group Population Health Initiative: Ambulatory Intensive Care Unit, PACE (Program for the All-Inclusive Care of the Elderly), the Veterans Health Administration Home-Based Primary Care Program, the largest value-based program in the country as well as with a private equity backed value-based visiting physician/home care program. His leadership focuses on collaborative interprofessional patient-centered development enhancing quality of care for high-risk patients. Dr. Vaidya is founder and CEO of Change Thinking Consulting, LLC providing interprofessional team coaching and consultation services. He is a Colonel in the Michigan Army National Guard with 20+ years of service including combat tours in Iraq and Afghanistan. He resides in Ann Arbor, Michigan, with his wife and two daughters, though in the summer you are more likely finding him at his family cottage on the lake in northern Michigan.

Preface

Congratulations on purchasing 9 *Essentials for Quality Health Outcomes in Older and High-Risk Patients: An Interprofessional Handbook*. First, commend yourself on your goodness within. Of the millions of choices of occupational fields, only a select few dedicate themselves in service and betterment of others. Thank you for purchasing this book. I am so privileged that highly regarded interdisciplinary professionals such as yourself place their confidence in this book. 9 *Essentials* empowers readers with a blueprint for successfully managing challenging patient complexity with compassion for the patient and the care team. You will find their application a watershed moment in your value-based journey. The 9 Essentials are actionable strategies with practical problem-solving insights for better care. They are holistic care, vital for physicians, nurses, physical and occupational therapists, dieticians, advanced practice providers, social workers, pharmacists, front-line workers, and mental health professionals. Health care executives reading this book find value in the 9 Essentials in empowering systems with improved outcomes and financial gains. I'm privileged, over the years, working in multiple health care settings in various roles. At each level, I've seen well-intentioned individuals get stuck, losing sight of how to be successful. This is particularly magnified as patient complexity increases. How would your interprofessional team address a verbally threatening patient with chronic pain driving exceptionally high emergency department utilization? What about a patient with dementia and frequent falls? Or even a medically complex patient who lands himself in the emergency department frequently while on alcohol intoxication binges?

Most teams struggle with cases like these, lacking tangible improvements. This book, among its many illustrated real-life patient case examples, walks you through each of these scenarios—how to approach, engage the interprofessional team, and produce results that are replicable in other complex patient cases. Healing occurs through thinking change. This book highlights how thought change at the interpersonal, individual, team, patient, and systems levels is crucial for improved health outcomes. As you read, you will encounter familiar topics, but also new and unique concepts and terms becoming part of your complex care vernacular. The book strikes a unique balance of didactic information, patient examples, and interactive reflection. Readers will find humor, inspiration, engaging stories, enlightening problem-solving, and humility. You will find *9 Essentials* a joy to read.

Why is *9 Essentials* important now? Health care is changing, with movement to value-based care. Plain and simple: Care aimed at better health outcomes is superior care. After decades of fee-for-service care, the US health care system is finally realizing this truth and tying outcomes to payment. In the United States, two federal changes, one a Republican initiative, the other a Democratic one, shifted health care payment structure. Medicare Advantage, the partial privatization of Medicare[1], and the Patient Protection and Affordable Care Act 2 introduced value-based purchasing to Medicar and Medicaid[2]. Health care systems find value-based reimbursement lucrative. When done right, the payout is higher than fee-for-service. Competition abounds among private health care start-ups, affordable care organizations, venture capitalists, and population health divisions. However, most value-based or at-risk programs have narrow margins for success. Much has been written on value-based care over the last decade. Many sources in population health exist describing data analytic tools and identifying at-risk patients, models of care, outcome measures, and clinical algorithms. The key is managing an at-risk cohort. Most health care institutions and programs struggle with providing meaningful, lasting patient outcomes because they lack knowledge and skills in the day-to-day interprofessional management of complex patients. Too often, interprofessional teams get stuck in a helpless state. Well-intentioned teams are unaware of their fatalistic approach, essentially giving up and saying, "There is nothing more we can do". This book details how approaching differently, with collaborative intellectual curiosity, unlocks helplessness for success no matter how challenging the complexity. The 9 Essentials of quality outcomes are illustrated through experience, case examples, and research. This, my friends, is where *9 Essentials* provides the tools to success. It is a down-to-earth, common-sense approach that does not overload with theory, statistics, charts and graphics, or pie-in-the-sky conjecture. If you can *change thinking*—this book speaks to you, enlightening your path and empowering care.

Patients' desires in health care are changing too. The largest growing segment of the health care population in the United States is the generation known as the baby boomers. This generation, the one of the Beatles and Woodstock, are progressive thinkers. They want individualized, convenient, timely care. Post-pandemic, more people want care in their home and not in a hospital or nursing home, with a greater desire for home-based services including virtual care and telehealth. Any successful program needs inclusion of these elements.

My journey began as a hospitalist including overseeing an intensive care unit in a small-town hospital following internal medicine residency. I found it very frustrating. The same patients cycled in and out of the hospital. As I tried problem solving, I was repeatedly told it did not have a role in inpatient care. I mostly heard "the patient is noncompliant" and is not going to change behaviors that landed them in the hospital. This did not align with my patient care philosophy. When my system started an ambulatory intensive care model, I jumped at the opportunity, designing interventions, reducing medical utilization and cost of care, and improving patient outcomes. This is where I began developing care interventions and honing them with real tangible results working for a program for the all-inclusive care of elderly (PACE) and later at a value-based VA home-based primary care program. This journey certainly was not linear, with difficult lessons along the way. I wrote this book first and foremost for imparting knowledge of what I learned and saw work for the betterment of both patients and providers. In my experience working in various settings, I've seen well-intentioned interdisciplinary professionals struggle with patient impacts, leaving them highly dissatisfied and professionally unfulfilled. Working through the 9 Essentials changes that. I developed them through insight—better patient outcomes develop through strong interdisciplinary team dynamics and a humanistic patient approach.

Most of the tenets of the nine principles are not natural to me. Because I work at them, I have better ability in communicating with others. Leadership and team building developed through the school of hard knocks for me. My career struggled. I am a natural introvert and from a young age struggled with interpersonal relationships. This followed me in my professional career. When a member of the AICU team verbalized giving up on a challenging, complex patient, I scolded them and called them out in front of the team. The team member was so distraught she filed a complaint with HR action. Several months later this team member took her own life. I live with the fact that my interaction negatively impacted someone already struggling. The 9 Essentials now provide a framework for complex patient problem-solving. I often think of this team member and am grateful for a better path forward when similar patient care frustrations arise.

In addition to interpersonal communication, my job performance, measured by patient satisfaction scores, was low. Measured outcomes such as utilization rates and cost of care followed. Patients were not following the prescribed intervention. I had three pivotal moments in my journey: (1) patient communication training, (2) team member mentorship, and (3) an unsuccessful medical directorship. My same interpersonal struggles with co-workers also occurred with patients. My patient satisfaction scores were abysmal. Unfortunately, this was common for providers during this era. Fortunately, my health system recognized a need and responded. They developed a focused education program consisting of both didactic and direct patient interaction observation focused on agenda setting, active listening, and empathy. As a concrete thinker, I found the material resources and experiential learning highly valuable skills I use to this day and have incorporated into 9 *Essentials*.

As you'll discover later in the book, today I recognize interpersonal connection is the most important part of life. This realization did not come naturally for me, coming later in life. This would not have happened if not for the guidance I received from my social work co-worker in the AICU. I credit her for guiding my thinking, transforming my clinical practice and outcomes. She is the most empathetic person I have ever met. She feels what patients feel, often sharing in their suffering and in their triumphs. Her advocacy for patients transformed my thinking. I began seeing patients' emotional as well as their physical needs. Subsequently my approach shifted away from systematic history taking to conversations. I began treating patients as individuals, learning about them as people, responding to empathy cues, and forming deeper connections. Patients began sharing their vulnerabilities. Soon they gained more trust, compliance went up, and outcomes improved. It was transformational for my clinical professional career- moving from frustration to highly rewarding.

Essential 3 (Check Your Ego at the Door) and Essential 4 (You Cannot Do It Alone) are revelations learned the hard way. After just over a year as medical director overseeing primary care of six centers in a rapidly growing value-based program, I stepped down. Utilization and medical cost of care were at an all-time high for the organization. The climate among the medical providers demonstrated poor morale with multiple interpersonal conflicts and overall poor job performance. I stayed on as a primary care physician and watched the new leadership transform key metrics seemingly overnight by engaging, listening, and resetting with the providers. It was a powerful lesson: Team dynamics through leadership are paramount for patient care success.

I wrote 9 *Essentials* for you—the health care interdisciplinary professional. You—physical therapist, dietician, occupational therapist, speech pathologist. You—nurse, advanced practice provider, pharmacist, physician. You—the health care administrator, executive, CEO. You—the health care bus driver, medical assistant, nursing aide, patient care technician. 9 *Essentials* demonstrates why all members of the team are key for success. Interdisciplinary teams are better when each interprofessional member thinks across disciplines. As you read, pay most attention to areas outside of your area of expertise.

The 9 Essentials were born out of trials and tribulations. I learned many lessons of leadership the hard way, but I also saw extraordinary patient successes in patient encounters like Kit Kline and Mr. Rodriguez, described in this book. The 9 Essentials impart how to do it easier. I want better for you, the reader. John Maxwell, an inspirational speaker and spiritual leader, talks about the "Law of Explosive Growth" and "Law of Legacy."[3] My hope is spreading knowledge and improving care on a large scale for both large numbers of patients and interdisciplinary professionals alike. *9 Essentials* empowers readers with essential tools for exponential spread.

With advancing age and increased number of chronic illnesses, palliative management is more appropriate than specialty or specialized procedural-based care. Primary care providers are trained in a wide spectrum of disease management. Fee-for service reimbursement dictated shorter visits with greater numbers of daily patient encounters. With limited time, practice shifted to specialty management. The difficulty is specialist care is not designed or equipped in follow-through care (visit frequency, access, etc.). The result is fragmented care across multiple specialties and multiple providers; not to mention increased cost for specialty visits. Ask yourself: How many times has a patient come back from a specialty visit with absolutely no change in management? Quality primary care is paramount in this patient population. The primary care team should oversee care, thereby reducing care fragmentation. Smaller panels open more availability for increased frequency of visits, acute care access, follow-up, goals of care, and end-of-life conversations. In addition to increased visit frequency, extended office visits allow more time for primary care management, reducing unnecessary specialty utilization. Early primary care follow-up following ED utilization or hospitalization is also key for readmission prevention.

The 80/20 rule states 80% of health care expenditures are on 20% of the population. More recent data suggests more than 80% of health care costs are due to 20% of the population.[4] For successful impact, you must target the top 10–20%. Unfortunately, the best estimators identifying this high-risk subset predict utilization of 30–40% at best. Therefore, I don't take much stock on one indicator over another. The best approach is having elements of number of chronic diseases, co-morbid psychiatric illness, social determinants of health, frailty, recent ED/hospitalization/ nursing home utilization, polypharmacy, and history of falls. Once you have identified your target population, *9 Essentials* is the guide on how to deliver results. Whether you are the direct care provider, population manager, or health care executive leader, this book is for you.

As you read, you will gain insight and practical know-how on the 9 Essentials of quality outcomes. How do you motivate a patient with frequent congestive heart failure exacerbations with poor primary care engagement and disease-specific counterproductive behaviors? What is your most important limitation standing in your way of success? How do you motivate an unmotivated team for success? What is most important to the patient? In life? How about a few pearls: How to manage a controlling patient or a frequent COPD exacerbator on maximal therapy? These and much more are found in the pages ahead. I am excited for you in this leap in your quest for better care and outcomes—full steam ahead!

References

1. H.R. 2015, Balanced Budget Act of 1997. Public Law No. 105-33. 1997.
2. H.T. 3590, Patient Protection and Affordable Care Act. Public Law No. 111-148. Washington, D.C.: 2009–2010.
3. Maxwell, J. C. *The 21 Irrefutable Laws of Leadership.* Nashville: Harper Collins, 2007.
4. Nash, E., Bethke, M., & Abrams, K. *The 80/20 Rule: Is It Still True? And What Can It Tell Us About 2018 and Beyond.* New York: Deloitte, 2018.

Acknowledgments

Mark Sasscer. You gave me inspiration for this book. When one door closed, you opened another one and guided me through it; I will never forget it.

Bruce Muma. You saw something in me before I realized it myself, starting me in my value-based care journey.

Mageada Mohamed. By example, you taught me what care is. Your support means more than words can ever express.

Kim Hurme. You made me a better doctor, guiding me to my empathy within.

Emily Hinske. Your depth instrumentally guided the path to publication. I am forever indebted.

Gwen Graddy. Thank you for naturally demonstrating and guiding humanistic values, enriching this book in so many ways.

Copyeditor Daniel Nighting. Your talent smoothing out the sharper edges of prose were invaluable improvements to the book.

Dissertation Editor Agent: Marquita Hockaday. Without your insights and industrious advocacy, publication would not have been possible.

Shivangi Pramanik and many others at CRC Press who's tireless work made publication a reality.

My many educators from years past at Greenhills School. Writing a book is only possible from the many lessons you gave me.

PART I

FUNDAMENTALS

CHAPTER 1

Essential 1: No One Is beyond Help

After just over a year as medical director, once again I returned to clinical practice at the same center I once directed. I found myself standing outside the door of the most well-known patient in the organization—Kit Kline. Kline was well known because she had the highest ED utilization of any patient across our very large value-based program. Kline went to the ED several times a week, and on occasion more than once on a single day. The previous physician at this site, tasked with meeting utilization quality metrics, grew tired of seeing her site "in the red" month after month. As medical director, I oversaw utilization metrics for the entire organization. If one or two sites struggled significantly, it had devastating effects on the company's annual metric goal and bottom line.

As you can imagine, as medical director, I was quite aware of Kit Kline. I sat in multiple meetings with her care team, coached her doctor on approaches to her management, even took frantic calls from her physician expressing her frustration and burn-out. The team employed various interventions with Kline to no avail. In fact, the more interaction with Kline, the more she went to the ED.

DOI:10.1201/9781003655084-2

Kit Kline unfortunately, like many Americans, suffered from chronic pain. She enrolled in our program on narcotic medication and eventually weaned down with the aid of the pain service specialist. However, Kline continued reporting chronic back pain. The clinic's narcotic contract required Kline submit serial urine drug screens. Despite prescribing her narcotics, multiple dosing a day, her urine showed no trace of narcotics. Her doctor stopped narcotic prescribing due to concerns of diversion (illegal distribution). Kline began acting out. She continued presenting to the clinic for scheduled and unscheduled visits, demanding pain management. This usually followed with presentation to the ED.

Kline's behaviors escalated, with her shouting demands at staff and her physician. She made threatening statements of harm toward herself and others, leading to multiple attempts at involuntary hospitalization for safety and concerns for self-harm. These were often unsuccessful due to her retractions of these statements at presentation to the ED. Various behavioral health medications were attempted; unfortunately, Kline would not take the medication. The behavioral health specialist diagnosed an axis II personality disorder, recommending setting and enforcing boundaries. Unfortunately, Kline began calling her social worker and case manager several times a day, often reporting issues needing immediate attention such as chest pain or suicidal ideation, necessitating 911 and ED referral. Kline came to the clinic several times a week, some weeks daily, demanding to be seen immediately. She started calling the after-hours staff repeatedly with the same severe and time-intensive complaints. Questions arose about Kline's competence. Legal proceedings followed, finding she did have capacity.

As you might imagine, the staff was quite frustrated with Kit Kline. She consumed precious time and resources. Frustration became burn-out, then countertransference. Good, well-intentioned staff caregivers began losing objectivity with Kline. Her verbal threats led to a behavioral contract. This too was unsuccessful, culminating in a physical altercation with the physician. Discussions began about involuntary disenrollment from our program. Pandemic regulations limited these options. The safety plan put in place included notifying local law enforcement each time Kline was on premises.

So here I am at her door, in this environment, with this backdrop. If you've spent some time in patient care, you've known a Kit Kline. What was the outcome? What do you think is Kline's outcome? Are you, like her caregivers, giving up hope? What happened next, when I went through that door and met Kline, was transformational, dropping her utilization to near zero. We'll dive deeper into the how and why later, but first we need a richer depth of understanding of Essential 1. No One is Beyond Help.

Provider Impacts

The complex patient suffers. Imagine lifting a poor soul by giving them a feeling someone has not given up on them. No matter how bad it is, there's always a way to help. *When you are not seeing improvement, you have not found the barrier for mitigation.* Barriers to improved care can run deep. Later sections of this book outline a path with pointers to get you there. Remember, *when you are stuck, you have to regroup, apply critical thinking, and approach the problem from a different perspective.* It's most important not to give up. *If their interprofessional advocate gives up, how can one expect a patient to keep hope?* If the interdisciplinary professional gives up hope and effort, why would a positive outcome occur? Keep in mind, *perfection is not the goal.* Complex patients have multiple chronic conditions, often with one or more severe and uncontrolled. *The goal is not zero utilization.* The goal more often is reduced utilization, more quality of time at home with friends or family, and reduced suffering from disease burden. Do not get discouraged when utilization occurs; for some conditions, it is an inevitability. It's about getting to the minimal number of hospitalizations and stopping the preventable ones.

If physicians reading this believe somehow their level of professionalism excludes them from giving up on patients, consider this: A large national study of 794 primary care practices found most practices reported dismissing patients in the previous two years, over 70% of these practices dismissed patients for repeated missed appointments, and nearly 50% dismissed patients for repeatedly not following health care recommendations.[1]

Patient Effects

Chronically ill patients get stuck. What I mean is they develop counterproductive thinking. Esteemed 20th-century cognitive psychiatrist Aaron Beck described *automatic thoughts—thoughts learned through habitual repetition occurring without conscious effort.* Beck described negative automatic thoughts causing behavioral pathology. For the complex patient, automatic thoughts such as, "I will never get better," "I am a burden to my family," "I am not a productive member of society," "I can't do anything," or "I am better off dead" produce self-defeating behaviors. Patients become more sedentary and often back away from prescribed treatments because they begin thinking nothing helps. Beck theorized automatic thoughts set up depression and anxiety disorders. Beck is considered a founding father of modern *cognitive-behavioral therapy (CBT)—uncovering irrational automatic thoughts, retraining thinking, and changing behavior to reinforce healthy thoughts.*

Patients with habitual negative thinking concerning their chronic disease often develop clinical depression. Chronic medical complexity and co-morbid depression have poorer clinical outcomes.[2] Often, those with self-defeating behaviors die sooner of their medical conditions, and unfortunately some take their own life. Depression requires identification and appropriate management. Aaron Beck also developed a depression screening tool known as the Beck Inventory of Depression (BDI). Today, inventories such as the PHQ-9 and cohort-specific tools such as the Geriatric Depression Scale (GDS) are more commonly used than the BDI because of ease and efficiency of use. Screen all complex chronic condition patients for depression frequently. Begin management early, utilize the primary team as much as possible, and refer to behavioral services when indicated. Patients often trust their primary care providers most. Managing complex patients requires rudimentary understanding of depression diagnosis, medical management, and CBT. Recognize your own deficits in these skills, seeking out further training through continuing education. The return on investment for your patients is extraordinary. Because of mental health stigma, many patients are reluctant for treatment and a basic start, from a trusted professional is a bridge to eventual acceptance of treatment. The bottom line is that automatic thoughts, self-defeating health behaviors, and clinical depression drive poor outcomes in older and chronically ill patients. For patients, *change thinking*—no one (even them) is beyond help.

Learned Helplessness

My undergraduate major was psychology. I had the great opportunity of studying under and working with the late Christopher Peterson at the University of Michigan on explanatory style, expectations, and depressive symptoms.[3] Peterson, along with Martin Seligman and Steven Maier, defined the theory of learned helplessness: repeated bad events perceived with lack of control leads to paralysis or helpless behavior.[4] Seligman first described learned helplessness in the 1960s with his work with groups of dogs. One group received an electric shock stimulus. The stimulus caused discomfort but did not have lasting damage. I am a firm believer that research with animals must be humane and just. If they pushed a lever, the shock stimulus ceased. Another group received the stimulus with no lever and could not stop the shock stimulus. Both groups of dogs were then placed in a new environment where they had to push down a divider to stop the shock. The group that could previously control the shocks learned quickly how to stop the shock in the new environment. The dogs who previously could not control the shock simply laid down when the stimulus was delivered in the new environment and never attempted pushing over the divider.[5]

Unfortunately, highly skilled health care providers commonly experience learned helplessness in caring for patients. They work tirelessly because of their cardinal truth that all health care providers want to help patients, seemingly without producing desired outcomes. They begin believing this is outside of their control. They develop learned helplessness in the form of intellectual paralysis, and like the dog receiving a shock stimulus, begin believing they no longer can change the outcome. Over the years I've seen this in many multidisciplinary care teams because of low success rates with high-risk patients. To some degree, every great team has elements of this phenomenon. Much like Seligman's dog in paralysis in a new environment it can control, your team too is likely stuck. Applying the 9 Essentials breaks this cycle. As a budding scholar of the 9 Essentials, you must help lead your team through the emblematic divider barrier.

Critical Thinking

Various models in critical thinking exist. Lean methodology describes the 5 Why's.[6] Like an inquisitive four-year-old, asking why to each answer refines specificity. The Institute for Healthcare Improvement's (IHI's) 4 Ms is another helpful tool.[7] The 4 Ms set a framework for analyzing complex cause and effect. Later versions add the fifth M for Co-Morbidity (Figures 1.1 and 1.2).

Whether you use the 5 Why's, 4 Ms, or another method is immaterial. What's important is getting to the root cause. A threat to critical thinking is judgment. Preconceived perceptions about patients sink the team's ability for getting to deeper levels of etiology. Notions stemming from narcotic use, criminal past, mental illness, socioeconomic status, gender, weight, race, and alcohol or drug use threaten the fidelity that no one is beyond help. This is magnified by group think. Redirect judgment thoughts or

Utilization 5 Why's

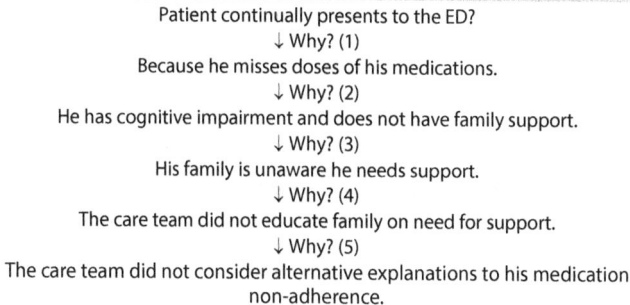

Patient continually presents to the ED?
↓ Why? (1)
Because he misses doses of his medications.
↓ Why? (2)
He has cognitive impairment and does not have family support.
↓ Why? (3)
His family is unaware he needs support.
↓ Why? (4)
The care team did not educate family on need for support.
↓ Why? (5)
The care team did not consider alternative explanations to his medication non-adherence.

FIGURE 1.1 Utilizing the 5 Why's in Determining the Root Cause of a Patient's High Emergency Department Visit Frequency.

5 Ms

Matters Most
What is most important to the patient (family)?
Mentation
What is their cognitive ability? Do deficits exist?
Medicine
Are there drug interactions, side-effects, or adherence issues?
Movement
Are there drug interactions, side-effects, or adherence issues?
Co-**M**orbidity (5th M)
What chronic disease states are contributing?

FIGURE 1.2 The 5 Ms Assessment of High-Risk Care.

statements into questions—ask why, how, what am I missing, what else is at play, how can I approach it differently?

Case Examples

Preventable Fall

A patient with dementia is brought to an adult day program via a patient transport bus. While staff assist non-ambulatory (wheelchair-bound) patients off the bus first, our patient with dementia becomes impatient and gets off the bus unattended. While walking from the bus into the center, she loses her balance, falls, and strikes her head. Undoubtedly, she is sent to the ED for head imaging. Upon her utilization review, her interdisciplinary team asks whether this was preventable, and what measures should be put in place for prevention in the future. Post-pandemic staffing shortages make adding staff for assistance off the bus not a reality. What to do to prevent a similar incident in the future? The team concludes this type of fall is not preventable. Are they correct? How would you proceed?

Because of her dementia, she is impulsive, increasing her fall risk. So, are falls an inevitability? What can possibly be done for mitigation? Upon first assessment, the team felt this was not preventable. They expressed frustration regarding short staffing. Likewise, the team felt *carry burden*—carrying the weight of ensuring patient safety in the setting of reduced resources magnified secondary to the patient also experiencing harm. Carry burden leads to feelings of guilt, defensiveness, and *intellectual paralysis*—one-way thinking without a solution or resolution. In this case, the team grappled with the fact that the limited staff prioritized movement of the non-ambulatory patients first. They believed the patient with dementia's fall was happenstance—one time behavior, exiting the bus unaccompanied with unsteady gait.

A team member began asking questions. Why did she try to exit the bus? Various disciplines contributed answers based on their expertise of dementia. With cognitive decline, behavior motivations become basic: When a bus comes to a stop at a destination, you exit the bus. A cognitively intact individual assimilates more information: location (is this your destination?) or taking direction to remain on the bus until another cue (the person ahead of you exists, a staff member directs you to later exit, etc.) For someone with dementia, they are cued by the bus pulling into a destination as a time for exit. For various physiological reasons, with cognitive decline, complex information processing is impaired; so too are short-term memory and inability remembering directions to remain on the bus. Further, frontal lobe degenerative changes diminish reasoning capacity, leading to impulsivity. The team began realizing there was a high probability for her behavior: wanting to exit the bus prior to staff availability for safe departure. Now let's address the carry burden with reassurance: The goal is not assigning blame; the goal is collaboration of critical thinking on causality for a future prevention. Accidents happen despite best practices. Once the team's feelings of guilt and fear of reprisal were openly discussed, the tension in the room melted away. The team became empowered. Courses of action directly addressing the patient's cognitions and tendencies began to flow. "Let's make sure she is the first one escorted off of the bus." "We'll make sure she is seated in the front of the bus. While we cannot have more staff on the bus, let's collaborate with the in-center staff for assistance helping her off the bus first upon arrival." On the surface, this case seems uncorrectable. With interdisciplinary in-depth evaluation, barriers and solutions are uncovered. Remember—*no one* is beyond help!

Let's Party

Another challenging case was Mr. Jay. Mr. Jay engaged in binge drinking. His favorite pastime was collecting his paycheck on payday and going out for the evening, walking (Mr. Jay did not have his own transportation) to one of the inter-city local casinos. Mr. Jay could not or would not control his drinking at the casino. This led to falls, altered mental status with loss of consciousness episodes, and questionable seizure-like activity. Every payday he went to the casino, thus turning into an EMS trip to the ED. Like clockwork, Mr. Jay had ED utilization every two weeks. Multiple office visit conversations discussing the risks took place with Mr. Jay after ED visits. Mr. Jay was of sound mind and expressing this was his enjoyment and he had no desire to change. Again, the care team was frustrated. A form of intellectual paralysis began taking shape: *the resolute fallacy*— belief that an individual is unwilling to change their behavior. Intellectual paralysis began taking hold of the team; they began believing no intervention would change Mr. Jay's ED utilization. Some even began believing it was his freedom of choice for Mr. Jay's self-destructive behavior. How did the team find their way to the essential that no one is beyond help?

What if we leaned into the resolute fallacy that Mr. Jay's casino drinking was not going to change but also avoided intellectual paralysis that an intervention could not change the outcome? What if Mr. Jay could go to the casino, drink heavily, but remain safe and out of the ED? By refocusing thinking in this way, the team began brainstorming potential interventions. What if we programmed Mr. Jay's cell phone with numbers to commercial ridesharing companies in addition to our clinic after-hours line who could help support and direct? Who is Mr. Jay's social support, and can we partner with them, encouraging safety and potentially even monitoring his casino trips? Are there other community partners at the casino? Can we provide cab vouchers for a safe ride home? Soon a plan developed including communications access, transportation, and social support. Soon Mr. Jay began going to the casino and not ending in the ED. The team's intervention barrier for Mr. Jay was the assumption that drinking alcohol will always lead to the ED. *If it seems impossible, you have not identified the barrier. Use critical thinking techniques with your team. You'll be surprised at the successful interventions you develop!*

Chapter Summary/Key Takeaways

Both patients and interdisciplinary professionals must recognize no one is beyond help. Repeated adverse stimuli for both patients and those caring for them contribute to negative automatic thoughts, learned helplessness, and depression. Key elements in navigating past these barriers include the following:

- Screen all high-risk patients for depression. Become skilled in general depression management and refer when appropriate.

- When you are not seeing improvement, you have not identified the barrier.
- When you get stuck, approach from a different perspective.
- Many methods for critical thinking exist, including methods outlined later in the book. It's less important focusing on choice of method; what matters most is that you get to that deeper etiology following a structured approach.
- Provider expectations drive patient results.
- Learned helplessness is perceived lack of control of repeated bad events, leading to paralysis or helpless behavior.
- Intellectual paralysis, a form of learned helplessness, is one-way thinking without a solution or resolution and is a threat to positive outcomes.
- Carry burden is the weight of ensuring patients' safety in challenging circumstances when the risk of harm and actual harm exists. Carry burden leads to feelings of guilt, defensiveness, and intellectual paralysis. Upcoming sections of this book outline how to manage carry burden.
- The resolute fallacy, a form of intellectual paralysis, is the belief that an individual is unwilling to change their behavior. Reducing carry burden and intellectual paralysis, including the resolute fallacy, is the key to success via Essential 1: No one is beyond help.

9 Essentials Case Study—Essential 1

Mr. Rodriguez is a 97-year-old man with advanced dementia and frequent hospitalizations with ensuing functional decline. He is dependent on iADLs and some ADLs while living alone in his home of the last 60 years. His wife of 52 years passed away 8 years ago. Mr. Rodriguez has three older adult children, Marie, Anna, and Felipe. Marie, his eldest daughter, is his primary care giver.

Mr. Rodriguez is enrolled in a wrap-around service program for high-risk patients. The interdisciplinary team (IDT) identifies care deficiencies at home driving hospital utilization and recommends a more structured living environment including long-term nursing facility placement. Following multiple family meetings, hospitalizations, and subacute rehabilitation/extended care stays, Mr. Rodriguez always returns home; the cycle begins again. Attempts at maximizing home care services are unsuccessful due to acuity of care and deficiencies in family support. The team is burned out with numerous calls because of increasing acuity, requests for more hours, and increasing behavioral disturbances, including hostility and uncooperative behavior. The team expresses frustration: "despite repeated interventions, Mr. Rodriquez's family is not able to care for him, repeatedly bringing him back home when he is unable to live independently." The IDT requests discontinuation from the program for nonadherence to the treatment plan. "We have done all we can do; the family is unrealistic and will not place him in a nursing home where he belongs. Outpatient management for a patient requiring higher level care can never work and if they are unwilling to accept this, we can no longer provide our services."

What are some examples of the resolute fallacy?
Where do you see elements of carry burden?
Where do you see elements of learned helplessness?
How would you *change thinking*, refocusing the team
  back from paralysis to care?

Feedback: 9 Essentials Case Study—Essential 1

What are some examples of the resolute fallacy?
  Despite repeated family meetings and education,
  the family's behavior does not change, with the

same poor outcome. The IDT states they believe their behavior is not going to change.

Where do you see elements of carry burden?

Multiple family meetings occur outlining increased needs, ultimately recommending nursing home placement; however, following each hospital stay or subacute rehabilitation extended care stay, the patient always returns home, and the cycle begins again. Attempts at maximizing home care services available are unsuccessful, and the team is burned out with numerous calls requesting more hours, acuity, and behavioral disturbance with an uncooperative and hostile patient increasing in frequency. The team expresses frustration that the family is not able to care for the patient, and despite repeated intervention, they continue bringing him back home. We have done all we can do; the family is unrealistic and will not place him in a nursing home where he belongs. We can no longer provide our services.

The risk of harm with repeated hospitalization for the patient is great. This drives the IDT's sense of frustration, defensiveness, and intellectual paralysis.

Where do you see elements of learned helplessness?

"Outpatient management for a patient requiring higher level care can never work and if they are unwilling to accept this, we can no longer provide our services."

How would you *change thinking*, refocusing the team back from paralysis to care?

Calling out the elephant in the room acknowledges the team's frustration. Allow them to respectfully discuss how they are feeling. Encourage them on the strides they made. Point out a shared sense of common purpose in helping the patient and family.

Ask, what would happen if we did nothing? If they disenrolled, would the prognosis worsen? If not us, who will help them?

Have we exhausted all opportunities for engaging the family? What are we missing? What are the family's barriers to providing care support?

Reflection
Essential 1: No One Is beyond Help

- Are you getting desired outcomes? If not, can you approach it from a different perspective? How can you change your thinking around the problem? What methods of critical thinking should you employ? What are potential barriers to successful outcomes?
- Carry burden is the weight of ensuring a patient's safety when harm or risk of harm is great. Do your interprofessional team members exhibit carry burden? How do they exhibit it?
- Intellectual paralysis is one-way thinking without solution or resolution. The resolute fallacy is a form of intellectual paralysis, a belief that an individual is unwilling to change their behavior. Are you or your team experiencing intellectual paralysis or the resolute fallacy? Provide some examples. What methods for critical thinking could help move past it?

References

1. O'Malley, A. S. Patient Dismissal by Primary Care Practices. *JAMA*. 2017; 177(7): 1048–1050.
2. Katon, W. J. Epidemiology and Treatment of Depression in Patients with Chronic Medical Illness. *Dialogues in Clinical Neuroscience*. 2011; 13: 7–23.

3. Peterson, C., & Vaidya, R. S. Explanatory Style, Expectations, and Depressive Symptoms. *Personality and Individual Differences*. 2001; 31(7): 1217–1223.
4. Maier, S., & Seligman, M. Learned Helplessness: Theory and Evidence. *Journal of Experimental Psychology*. 1976; 105(1): 3–46.
5. Seligman, M. Learned Helplessness. *Annual Review of Medicine*. 1972; 23: 407–412.
6. Ohno, T. *Toyota Production System: Beyond Large-Scale Production*. Portland: Productivity Press, 1988.
7. *Age-Friendly Health Systems: Guide to Using the 4Ms in the Care of Older Adults*. New York: 2020.

CHAPTER 2

Essential 2: Right Care, in the Right Place, at the Right Time

Very dear to my heart is my love of my country. I'm not speaking about nationalism but about deep admiration for its founding essence of liberty, justice, and equality for all. My grandfather served in the Second World War. My grandmother supported the war effort on the home front, one of many women in the workforce, as manufacturing turned to the development of military equipment. My mother, a baby boomer, grew up in a post-war working-class family living the American Dream (having more than enough; happily living within their means). My father was an immigrant to this country. He made a choice: immigrating for life, liberty, and the pursuit of happiness. And in this great country, a foreign land for him, he started from little and prospered.

I always had a desire to serve my country. In college, I was not ready for this commitment but had a few friends in the Reserve Officers' Training Corps (ROTC). By the time I was in medical school, 9/11 occurred, and I was ready—taking a leap of faith, joining the Michigan Army National Guard as a commissioned officer. The year following completion of my residency training was eventful. In November

DOI:10.1201/9781003655084-3

I got married, and two months later I left my young bride at home, deploying in support of Operation Iraqi Freedom to Basra, Iraq. (Two years later I would deploy again, to Kabul, Afghanistan, and this time we were expecting our first child!)

There I was, barely six months out of training, a young physician tasked with practicing 21st-century medicine amid a warzone. In residency training I had every resource with an expectation to use it (whether I needed it or not). Practicing medicine in the Army, in a warzone, was different. Very few immediate supports existed outside of point-of-care blood testing, portable x-ray, and an EKG machine. Specialized care, including advanced imaging, was available, but there was a catch—it required patient movement. Movement across a battlefield is tricky. Yes, resources including fuel, supplies, and personnel are always at a premium. Patient movement for advanced care was risky and often dangerous due to enemy threats and environmental conditions like sandstorms threatening air movement. A unique risk not encountered in the US civilian health care system. Clinical decision-making involved asking: Is this trip necessary, i.e., will advanced testing or treatment alter the natural progression of disease? Is it worth the risk of medevac? It is not safe ordering unnecessary care. This situation forced me to make critical decisions: Whether the potential benefits of advanced treatment outweighed the risks.

This experience emphasized the importance of astute clinical skills—history-taking, observation, examination, and intuition—over extensive testing and interventions. It was a humbling experience, teaching me much of what is done in modern medicine can be unnecessary and even harmful. Trust me, I put many patients on those flights during my two tours of duty. There are circumstances warranting higher levels of care. As you decide on sending patients to a higher level of care, think of the *metaphorical mede-vac helicopter*—risk of moving a patient to a higher level of care. The equation for mitigating the risk of the metaphorical medevac helicopter = **The Right Patient + The Right Setting + The Right Time.**

Value-Based Care
Payment Structure

Accountable care organizations, as well as for-profit entities, see economic rewards of risk contracting—accepting upfront payment and mitigating costs. If the organization outspends it's a loss but if it under-spends, then the savings are kept. Of course, there are negotiated up-side and down-side risk arrange-ments on how each party shares in the cost and sav-ings. A very successful model is the Program for the All-Inclusive Care of the Elderly (PACE). PACE began in the 1970s in California, and the model quickly caught on. Its effectiveness in reducing health burden and costs eventually got support of the US Congress, passing Title 42 US Code 1396u-4: Program of All-inclusive Care for Elderly (PACE),[1] allocating individ-uals' Medicaid dollars to PACE programs as capitated payments with full risk. The PACE program in a sense acts as managed care. When costs are less than capitated payment, it is reinvested into the program; however, when costs exceed revenue, the program is at financial risk. The program works because of its wrap-around services including transportation, a day center with life enrichment activities, pharmacy, case management, home care, primary care, and nursing working in tandem for meeting PACE par-ticipants' needs. PACE realized years before today's value-based care movement that investing in meeting patient needs (including nonmedical needs such as adequate access to food and shelter) has great returns.

Other value-based payment structures include bundled payments tying payment to positive health outcomes, known as value-based purchasing. An under-rated payment structure is capitation—payments based on patient risk. For the Centers for Medicare and Medicaid Services (CMS), the United States's largest payer, payments are capitated. The nation's largest health care system, the Veterans Health Administration (VHA), realized economic benefits for capitated payments several years ago. Funding for the VHA occurs through annual congressional appropriations. Most of the funding for any individual Veterans Affairs Medical Center (VAMC) occurs through the Veterans Equitable Resource Allocation (VERA).[2] VERA dollars are determined by the need of each VAMC. Hospitals with higher acuity veterans receive more funding. In many ways the VHA were ahead in value-based care, establishing home-based primary care (HBPC) several years before most health care systems developed dedicated programs for high-risk primary care patients.

HBPC provides multidisciplinary care including primary care, pharmacy, rehabilitation, psychology, social work, nursing, and nutrition in the veteran's home for those most at risk of poor health outcomes. The model is highly successful in reducing health burden and reducing hospital utilization cost.[3] Even more remarkable, unlike other value-based programs aiming at cost reduction, HBPC generates revenue. Dedicated time and resources in a high-risk population produce more robust documentation capture of multiple conditions, translating into more VERA funding.

CMS capitated payments and VERA dollars share a commonality: Both are government payments to health care systems based upon the acuity of the population they serve. Like VERA, CMS assesses need based upon Hierarchical Condition Category (HCC) codes. HCC codes are weighted by condition complexity. Higher complexity codes or multiple conditions increase patient risk with higher CMS pay-out. Just like the VA HBPC Program, non-VA value-based programs can generate large returns through increased HCC capture.

Key Tenets of Value-Based Care

Care in the Right Setting: Paradigm Shift from Institutionalized Care to Care at Home

Fee-for-service ties reimbursement to in-person office visits, i.e., more visits means more billing. Getting out of the home can be physically not possible, too tasking, or improbable due to lack of adequate transportation in the chronically ill. A silver lining of the global COVID-19 pandemic came through greater ability for telemedicine care. In many instances, with good history, knowledge of the patient, in-home staff, or virtual assessment technology, patients can receive care and services at home. *Insisting on in-person clinic care can overburden patients and caregivers and erode trust.* Likewise, requiring in-center visits can delay care with patients deteriorating while arranging transportation.

A couple years ago, we took a family road trip. In anticipation, I called the local mechanic and asked if my vehicle was due for preventative maintenance for reducing the risk of a breakdown on the long car trip. I provided my make, model, and mileage. The office staff said only a certified mechanic could give advice and suggested I bring the vehicle in to look over. I took time off work and scheduled the visit. I parked out front, checked in, and awaited my inspection. I watched as my truck sat still, parked in view out the window. After about 15 minutes the receptionist came to me and said the mechanic had looked things over and I was not due for preventative maintenance. I asked how he came to that conclusion because my vehicle never left its parking space. She said he looked up the information on the computer. I asked why he couldn't do that when I first called and avoided the unnecessary trip in? She was speechless. The dumbfounded look she gave me summed up the shop's operations. It's not customer-centric. In fact, the viewpoint of the customer was not even considered. I never went back to that mechanic shop. *Patients trust you will only inconvenience them for essential care. Don't bring patients in for care that can be delivered over the phone, computer, or in the home.*

Another key lesson from the pandemic—care in the home with family and other social supports is preferred over institutionalized care. Isolation restrictions and health care staffing shortages made hospitals and nursing homes undesirable. Preferences for receiving care in the home continued beyond the pandemic with an explosion of in-home care services.[4]

Care Stewardship

Just as unnecessary office visits are burdensome, so too is unneeded testing. Testing should occur if it will change management and improve care. Most medically complex patients are in palliative stages. Tests and procedures that do not provide long-term benefit, are overly burdensome to patients and families, or have risks of further harm (remember the metaphorical medevac helicopter) should be avoided. Start goals of care discussions early with patients and families. Educate on risks and benefits of aggressive care and end-of-life modalities (hospice, comfort measures) when appropriate. When discussing quality of life, I always consider: *There are things worse than death.* Everyone defines what is worse than death to them (artificial life support, nursing home confinement, etc.).

Unlike value-based care, fee-for-service incentivizes testing and procedures. Reimbursement is based on relative value units (RVUs), assigning dollar value to procedures and services. RVUs increase with increasing number of service encounters. Traditionally health care systems were set up for maximizing billable encounters for increased profits. Systems incentivize providers for increasing RVUs. Unfortunately, this often conflicts with patient needs, especially magnified in high-risk populations. Take for example colorectal screening through colonoscopy, a minimally low risk endoscope procedure. The risk/benefit ratio for colonoscopy is higher in complex and frail patients. Benefits such as increased longevity may not apply as they will likely succumb to existing conditions rather than live long enough for experiencing the burden of colon cancer. Furthermore, given a low functional baseline, treatment modalities such as surgery and chemotherapy may have worse outcomes in complex patients, not to mention complications arising from colonoscopy preparation (electrolyte imbalances with delirium, falls ensuing from trips to the bathroom) as well as transportation barriers for the procedure. Despite this, many health care providers are incentivized to recommend colonoscopy in this cohort, even in some cases penalized for not recommending the procedure. Value-based purchasing rewards good care by tying patient outcomes to reimbursement. Value-based programs have higher provider job satisfaction, not only because providers have care agency with improved outcomes but also because they work smarter, not harder. They are financially incentivized for their time spent in managing patient care over the number of patients seen. They are incentivized for quality care, not quantity of encounters, often with fewer but more meaningful encounters a day. Providers are more satisfied spending time taking care of their patients' needs rather than struggling fitting in time for meeting their needs.

Timing of Care

Chronic disease management requires frequent evaluations or touch points. Seeing the doctor once or twice a year will not meet patient needs. Make sure they are seen as appropriate. Anticipate acuity increases and get ahead of them by decreasing time between touch points. When changes occur unexpectedly such as an emergency room visit or hospitalization, see them soon after discharge. Increase frequency of visits following utilization for ensuring stability. Setting standards of frequency of follow-up based on acuity, utilization, or at the initiation of a patient to a value-based initiative helps ensure patients are seen at an appropriate touchpoint, at a frequency reasonable for the patient, so as not to create visit burn-out. Set reasonable panel sizes, allowing availability for frequent follow-up.

Access to Urgent Care

True emergencies—immediate threats to life, limb, or eyesight—belong in the emergency room. Urgent care—care that if delayed will lead to emergent care—should be managed outside of the ED. Risk of complications arises when urgent care is treated in an emergent setting. Chronically ill patients need 24-hour access to urgent care, whether it is an after-hours line, community paramedicine, or a free-standing clinic. Lower patient panels also facilitate better understanding of individual needs. It is much easier for a provider determining urgency versus emergency if the patient is well-known to the provider.

Individualize Care

Have you ever had a patient come back to you from the ED or hospital and say: "They didn't do anything for me"? Most often there is a disconnect in expectation. The patient is often looking for definitive management. A hospital, and certainly an emergency department, is set up for management of acute life-threatening conditions that cannot be managed on an outpatient basis. *Emergency medicine (in a nutshell) is asking—Is this going to kill them immediately? If so, I will treat now; if not, move them to more definitive care.* A common example is admission for chest pain (noncardiac). Once a cardiac etiology is ruled out, the patient is discharged. "But I still have the pain!" Most commonly the cause is gastrointestinal reflux disease. A thorough history on the quality of pain, with aggravating and alleviating symptoms, will likely get the patient to definitive management (again what they are looking for).

Let's look at the case of altered mental status in a patient with dementia. The patient presents to the ED, and work-up ensues. Clinical results show a slight increase of BUN/Cr, indicating dehydration and presence of bacteria in the urine without clear evidence of an inflammatory reaction. A diagnosis of metabolic encephalopathy with urinary tract infection is made. The patient is admitted to the hospital, going from ambulatory to non-ambulatory (except for the occasional trip to the bathroom or brief physical therapy session). After a day or two, functional ability decreases, and disposition becomes subacute rehabilitation (SAR) placement. SAR placement is generally a minimum of two weeks. While they are there for rehab, they are often less active than they would be at home. The patient comes out of the hospital/SAR experience with worse functional ability than they went in with. How can a patient go into a health care facility set up to improve health outcomes, yet come out worse? The answer is the risk of this metaphorical medevac helicopter ride (hospitalization) is too great—it is the wrong setting for care. Prompt work-up and outpatient management, especially in cases of negative findings, such as dementia education on cognition waxing/waning from moment to moment occurs commonly, often reassures and reduces caregivers' expectations in acute care settings. The lay public understands dementia as a degenerative process with cognitive decline. Less known is the fact that degenerative CNS changes lead to changes in mentation worsening over time. Fluctuations in the sleep–wake cycle and patient awareness are commonplace. Dementia is a progressive disease averaging about 10 years from short-term memory slips to being bed-bound with complete loss of functional ability, cumulating in death from pneumonia or other infective secondary processes. *Educate dementia caregivers that it's a mixture of "good days" (high alertness and functional ability) and "bad days" (low alertness and functional ability). Early in the condition's course there are more good days than bad. Later there are more bad days than good.* Bad days are part of the natural history of the disease process and not a mark of a secondary process. Because of this, treatment for a secondary process is not indicated. Therefore, providing care for a condition the patient does not need (such as a urinary tract infection), in the wrong setting, at the wrong time inevitably leads to poorer outcomes. Reassurance and supportive care at home have a better outcome (maintaining in a familiar environment with more activity) because the bad day will subside.

Unfortunately, the fee-for-service system leaves little time for thorough evaluation in primary care. Many conditions internists and family physicians are trained to manage, such as hypertension, diabetes, and heart failure, are referred out because of competing office demands. Specialty care also is high-volume challenged. Take for example Shayne Hillsborough, a patient with coronary disease and hypertension following with a cardiologist for management. He presents for an early-morning office visit with elevated blood pressure readings. The cardiologist increases his beta blocker, and the next day he starts the increased dose, has a syncopal episode, and falls and breaks his hip. What happened? The wrong care in the wrong setting. Routine hypertension is best managed in primary care because it is better set up for following blood pressure longitudinally, developing long-term patient relationships, and understanding psychosocial dynamics. Had Shayne Hillsborough presented to his primary care's office with elevated blood pressure, his primary care team, having more familiarity with his medication administration patterns, would more likely consider other causes of his elevated blood pressure such as missing his medications on hurried days when he has office appointments.

Chapter Summary/Key Takeaways

- Complex care management requires a value-based approach based on individualized care for the right patient, in the right setting, at the right time.
  - The metaphorical medevac helicopter is inappropriately sending patients to higher levels of care including specialty, emergency, hospital, imaging, and procedures placing patients at higher risks. Placing patients in the appropriate level of care mitigates these risks.
- Value-based care is a rising and lucrative market.
  - Value-based purchasing—bundled payments tie payment to positive health outcomes.
  - Capitation—payment based upon patient risk. Greater opportunities exist through CMS Capitated Hierarchical Condition Category (HCC) payments.
- Key tenets of value-based care include:
  - Care in the *right* setting
  - Care stewardship—care that is indicated; avoidance of unneeded care

- Timing—care *when* needed
- Access—to preventative and urgent care
- Increase care access through precision—care frequent enough for prevention, 24-hour access for exacerbations, and use of adjuvant technology such as virtual capabilities and monitoring.

9 Essentials Case Study—Essential 2

Marie Rodriguez Stanine, first born and the apple of her father's eye, was "Daddy's Little Girl." She always pined for her father's affection. Mr. and Mrs. Rodriguez immigrated to the United States in search of a more prosperous life from their ancestral home in a rural Mexican village. They both had no advanced education beyond high school. They immigrated during the automotive manufacturing boom of the 1960s. Mr. Rodriguez found well-paying, steady work at the Clark Street Assembly Plant in southwest Detroit, Michigan producing Cadillacs. He settled with similar immigrants in the inner-city neighborhood known as Mexican Town.

Like many factory workers of the time, Mr. Rodriguez desired higher education for his children with the hope they would be less reliant on manual labor occupations. Marie was the first in her family to graduate from college. She first obtained her associate degree as a registered nurse and eventually her bachelor of nursing. She worked med-surg at one of the inner-city hospitals. Marie focused on her education and career. She married later in life to a fellow med-surg nurse, eventually having three children of her own. She instilled her father's education values in her children, but only one of them completed college. Her youngest, Kathryn, struggled in school and in the workforce, remaining living at home. Her middle child, Sophie, became pregnant in high school.

The father fled the situation (which legally was easier to do in those days), leaving Marie's family strapped with the financial responsibilities of supporting her grandson, Thomas, in addition to the other members of the household.

Felipe Rodriguez was a tortured soul. As the only son, his father viewed him differently, with expectations the son would be in the father's likeness. However, they were different, often clashing. Felipe was closer to his mother, who showed him favoritism as the youngest and only boy. By upper elementary school he was a worrier, by junior high school he was diagnosed with anxiety, and by high school he was drinking heavily. He had difficulty keeping steady work secondary to his affliction for alcohol, which was often a point of contention with his father, who always held one steady job. Felipe's alcohol use disorder affected his interpersonal relationships, with two failed marriages and strained relationships with his children. His mother's terminal illness and death threw Felipe over the edge; what little control he had over his drinking was now lost. By the time of his father's decline, Felipe's health deteriorated into manifestations of liver failure vacillating between alcohol-induced encephalopathy and brief periods of clarity.

* * *

Anna walked from the facility to the car parked out front brought up by her husband. She carefully sat down in the passenger seat, and they drove off. Her cell phone rang. Staring back up at her, the screen identified the caller: Marie. Anna felt deflated having to take a call from her sister. She said to her husband, "I bet this is about Dad again." Anna answered, and Marie described how their father, currently hospitalized after yet another fall at home, is being discharged later that day.

The case worker at the hospital is adamant about him going to a nursing home. I just can't do that to him again, Anna. He's been in so many of them, and they're all terrible. He's never clean. He hates it there. He's always more confused in the nursing home. The only way they manage his outbursts is sedating him—then either he falls again, or they send him back to the hospital for confusion or some other reason. I don't know what to do. This is so hard. Making matters worse, Sophie's overtime was cut back, and little Tommy needs new school clothes. I'm having to pick-up some temp work to make ends meet. I don't want to burden you with this. I know you help as much as you can in your condition. I really didn't want to call you about this because I know you had chemo today, and that always takes so much out of you. I just really need some support again with the case worker. We want to take him home again, and you know Felipe is no help.

Anna sighed. She dreaded time after chemo. Already on the way home, she began feeling intense fatigue. All she wanted to do was go home and climb into bed. She felt for her sister. Anna also felt guilty as she would like to do more but is physically limited by the breast cancer that ravaged her body. It weighed on her, not much unlike her own mother, who succumbed to the same disease a decade earlier. Back then, Anna was very involved with her mom's care along with Marie and her father. Mrs. Rodriguez was a very devout Catholic. For Mrs. Rodriguez, her faith instilled in her preservation of life. This came into conflict when her disease process and advanced age made advanced treatment improbable. End-of-life decisions, including eventual enrollment into hospice, were delayed mainly because Mr. Rodriquez wanted to honor his wife's religious convictions, as much as he secretly wanted to make her more comfortable, especially when her cognitive function and competence slipped away in advanced metastatic disease.

Once again, Anna had to politely decline Marie's request to come to the hospital and participate in her dad's discharge planning.

Both Marie Rodriguez and the care team identify lapses in Mr. Rodriguez's care. The two are not in agreement on best management for Mr. Rodriguez.

How does the family describe inappropriate care? How does the care team?

Where is the team stuck? How can you approach the case differently?

Feedback: 9 Essentials Case Study—Essential 2

How does the family describe inappropriate care? How does the care team?

The family believes a nursing home is an inappropriate level of care. They feel it does not provide adequate care and is too restrictive, with loss of dignity. The family possibly believes they can provide adequate care at home, with a sense of guilt around placement. The care team cites increased care needs with lack of adequate support and resources in the home for Mr. Rodriguez's needs.

Where is the team stuck? How can you approach the case differently?

The team is stuck because the family and care team are striving for different goals. The care team, experiencing care burden, wants a structured living environment. The family's goals are mixed and in conflict—denial in terms of need, guilt/remorse, misperceptions of capabilities, financial strain, etc. Exploring patient and family goals is the first step in moving in a common direction with shared positive outcomes. We'll explore this more in Essential 6.

Reflection
Essential 2: The Right Care, in the Right Place, at the Right Time

- Are your patients receiving care in the right setting? Are they receiving care in a higher acuity setting than their needs dictate? What risks does this assume? How can you intervene in inappropriate escalation of care?
- How can you improve access to care after hours?
- How can you leverage technology in care delivery?

References

1. United States Code, Supplement 4, Title 42, Subchapter XIX, sec 1396u-4: Program of All-inclusive Care for Elderly (PACE). 2006 Edition.
2. Department of Veteran Affairs. *Veterans equitable resource allocation.* Washington, DC: Author, 1997.
3. Edes, T., & Kinosian, B. Better access, quality, and cost for clinically complex veterans with home-based primary care. *Journal of the American Geriatrics Society.* 2014; 62(10): 1954–1961.
4. Bestsennyy, O., & Chmielewski, M. *From Facility to Home: How Healthcare Could Shift by 2025.* Mckinsey & Company, 2022.

CHAPTER 3

Essential 3: Check Your Ego at the Door

Dr. A is a very learned and accomplished psychologist with a Ph.D. and clinical certification specializing in psychosis in the face of dementia. He is very well-intended, always having the patient's best interest at heart. Unfortunately, he believes because of his advanced training, he knows best. Dr. A leads his team's weekly case conference. He had his organization's standardized worksheet based on the 4Ms. With the interdisciplinary team (IDT) assembled in the meeting, Dr. A went through each section of the grid filling out each M on his own without input from the team. He made wide assumptions based on his vantage point. Dr. A became defensive with dissenting opinions from the team. This spilled over with him once telling a patient, "I know this treatment is best because I am a board-certified mental health specialist!" Interestingly the action plan section of Dr. A's worksheet lacked detail, specifics, and even completely empty sections because not every 4M conformed to psychological principles. Dr. A would remark: "Well there's nothing else we can do here."

DOI:10.1201/9781003655084-4

He felt this way because he was out of ideas (and in his mind only he could solve it). Dr. A never realized others may have ideas that work. Despite his best efforts, his team performed worst in utilization metrics across his organization. Why? Dr. A could not get out of his own way, suspend his ego, and empower diverse creative thinking.

Psychological Self-Concept

Sigmund Freud defined ego as the self's interaction with the outside world.[1] Freud described a set of defense mechanisms in the unconscious mind for protection from internal stress. His daughter, Anna Freud, later described defense mechanisms as unconscious resources used by the ego.[2] A more contemporary psychologist, George Kelly, described *personal construct theory (PCT)* in the mid-20th century. PCT contends individuals interpret the world around them through a set of hierarchical schemas or constructs. Constructs tend to have two poles such as good and bad. Dysfunction occurs when these constructs are in conflict, and interventions are aimed at rebuilding and rebalancing constructs.[3] Many experts believe PCT is the foundation of modern cognitive behavioral therapy. Under PCT, the self-construct is susceptible to distortion.

Combining Freud and Kelly, defense mechanisms are used by the ego for self-protection from internal strife when external stimuli directly conflict with the self-construct. The point of all of this is the ego is closely tied to our motivations and is continually threatened by external forces. Defense mechanisms exist for protection of the ego but are often in conflict with our goals. Now that you understand the workings of the ego, we'll next discuss how to check your ego at the door.

Get Out of Your Own Way

Health care professionals are just that—professionals. Health care professionals have advanced education, and in the case of physicians, doctorate and post-doctoral (residency) education. The global COVID-19 pandemic reinforced and strengthened societal esteem for this profession. There is also a well-deserved feeling with the work of helping others and improving lives. Fields managing life-and-death decisions (e.g., health care, law enforcement, military) are typically hierarchical, with tight command-and-control structure discouraging dissent from subordinates. All of this contributes to a positive ego and self-worth schema.

Care for the most complex patients requires analytical thinking. Health care, including training, is set up for a time long past, a time before longevity with chronic illness existed. A time when a fee-for-service delivery systems and 15-minute office visits worked. As the number of treatments expanded, medical education absorbed additional training. The outcome was linear education—cause and effect, diagnosis to treatment. Today, health care education curricula are more didactic. Working outside one's norms, thinking different from training and experience, and receiving input from other disciplines, creates internal stress and threatens ego. Defense mechanisms go up, and pursuit of better care stifles.

Suspending your ego also means relinquishing control. Complex management requires critical thinking from an interdisciplinary team. This cannot occur in a command-and-control environment. As physicians, we are used to having control, the last say, and in certain medical situations it is appropriate, but for the most part, in complex care management it is not. The team functions when it is a team of equals because no discipline is more important in finding the solution. This is often where most interventions fail: placing the medical professional at the top, with preference for a medical solution to a psychosocial problem. The PACE model has a proven success track record with national growth and expansion. The core of its success rests on the foundation that the 11 members of its interdisciplinary team are equal. The physician is no more important than the bus driver because the driver sees the inside of a participant's home, observes their mobility on and off the bus, develops a rapport from the frequent and often daily contact, and observes subtle changes before a case manager call or a provider visit. Empowering the driver brings key information forward for management.

We've discussed conscious efforts in suspending one's ego, but as Freud identified, the ego is an unconscious phenomenon. Freud theorized 10% of human motivation and behavior is conscious to the mind whereas 90% is unconscious and unaware to the individual. We extrapolate in modern-day human communications that most human communication is non-verbal (unconscious) occurring through unconscious cues or body language. Today, thanks to the work of researchers John Mayer, Peter Salovey,[4] and psychologist Daniel Goleman,[5] emotional intelligence helps bridge this gap. *Emotional intelligence is the ability to recognize and manage your own emotions while appropriately responding to the emotions of others.* Recognizing our unconscious communication with others, our self-concept and perceived influence over others, as well as others' nonverbal communication, is foundational for a willingness for working as equals.

Cardinal Truth

One of the best team exercises in health care is sitting down together and asking each member of your care team why they got into this field. It's so power-ful because it surfaces the *cardinal truth: Health care providers enter their field for altruism.* Talking about everyone's cardinal truth highlights shared values, which are unifying. Table 3.1 outlines threats to the cardinal truth.

TABLE 3.1   Threats to the Cardinal Truth

Cardinal Truth Threat	Mechanism	Example
Ego	Altruism gives way to power and self-worth	*The self interacting with environment:* Influenced by ■ Freudian defense mechanisms ■ Emotional intelligence *Personal construct theory:* Individuals interpret the world around them through a set of hierarchical schemas or constructs. *Emotional Intelligence:* The ability to recognize and manage your own emotions and recognize and appropriately respond to the emotions of others.
Burn-out	Self-destructive behaviors replace altruism due to competing priorities	*Work–life balance:* High workloads and diminishing returns, leading to lackadaisical paralysis and priorities shift away from care outcomes to outside priorities (i.e., family obligations).
Greed	Selfishness replaces altruism	*Fee-for-service:* Monetary compensation overtakes pursuit of great care. Compensation increases with more billable services such as numbers of patient encounters, testing, and procedures.

Case Examples
I Don't Trust You

Wally Gustoff is a recluse, more comfortable in solitude. Because of his experience with fragmented care in the health care system, he is very mistrustful of clinicians. Unfortunately, Mr. Gustoff suffered from decompensated heart failure and chronic back pain secondary to multi-level spinal stenosis. He desired a curative surgery for his back pain, seeing multiple specialists, including neurosurgery and cardiology, and undergoing multiple testing modalities with the conclusion: Wally is medically too high risk for spinal decompression surgery. Despite conservative management, his pain persisted. He became more mistrustful of the medical community as he viewed: "they're holding me from my surgery." Wally turned inward, nursing his woes with salty food. The team realized he was headed for a catastrophic congestive heart failure exacerbation. He was resistant to any in-clinic or virtual visit intervention. What to do?

The team realized more time in the day program gave more opportunities for monitoring and intervention. The barrier was Mr. Gustoff's rapport with the clinical team. An interdisciplinary team member connected some of the dots. The community health center had a jetted tub, mostly used for calming effects for patients with dementia. The team member realized the jet tub buoyancy, warm water, and soothing jets might offer back pain relief in addition to being a great patient satisfier, gaining greater trust with him and associating a positive outcome with the team's prescribed intervention. It likewise provided an opportunity for Mr. Gustoff to be in the center frequently for closer observation and rapport building. Eureka! By stifling others' thoughts, this type of out-of-the-box solution could not be sought.

They're Out to Get Me!

Darren Shine, an elderly man with complex chronic disease managed through a high-risk patient program, lives in an inner-city housing unit. Adjacent housing units in his building had an outbreak of bed bugs. Mr. Shine refused access to his unit as part of regulatory surveillance and mitigation, stating, "They are out to get me!" The IDT was perplexed. Members of the IDT had been in the patient's home and did not suspect bed bug manifestation spread there. Why was he so concerned? One of the team members thought it might be because of the urine odor from the multiple filled urinals around his apartment. Why was Mr. Shine using urinals? Was it a hardship walking to the bathroom? The rehab therapist stated Darren Shine had no mobility concerns and did not require assistive mobility devices. As the team explored further, the rehab therapist became defensive: "I've been doing this a long time, I've assessed his gait, he has no difficulty walking and should have no concerns making it to the bathroom." In many situations, the inquiry often stops here.

"Can we get another in-home assessment?" said another IDT member. "What about his bathroom? Is it functioning for him, plumbing, etc.? Are there barriers to mobility in the bathroom?" At this point, the rehab specialist, embodying his professionalism, suspended his ego and agreed to another in-home assessment. This time he assessed Mr. Shine's navigation of his bathroom. Because of his enlarged prostate, Mr. Shine had difficulty initiating and controlling his urine stream, finding it more conducive sitting on the toilet to void. The rehab therapist observed Mr. Shine had significant difficulty getting up and down from the toilet, and the therapist recommended a toilet riser and wall grab bars. Additionally, the assessment afforded an opportunity for interdisciplinary collaboration with the physician for managing Mr. Shine's prostatic hypertrophy affecting his micturition. Mr. Shine was so gracious for the intervention that significantly reduced the hardship and improved his quality of life. When we realize it's not about us or our expertise, it's always about patient betterment, great things are possible!

Chapter Summary/Key Takeaways

Keys for success include the ability for self-reflection and understanding you are not the most important person in the room. It appears a simple concept on the surface but is very challenging in practice. Identifying and addressing the following will help you achieve success:

1. *The cardinal truth*: Health care providers enter the field to help others. Once you realize this commonality it's easier giving folks a seat at the Table 3.2. Embrace the cardinal truth; leverage its power in empowering others. Threats to the cardinal truth and mitigation strategies include the following.

TABLE 3.2   Mitigating Threats to the Cardinal Truth

Threats to Cardinal Truth	Mitigation Strategies
Ego: Self-importance can overshadow altruism, leading to power struggles and reduced team effectiveness.	**Reaffirm altruistic motives**: Regularly remind team members of their core motivations.
Burn-out: High demands and stress can shift focus away from patient care to personal survival.	**Support work–life balance**: Address factors contributing to burnout to maintain focus on patient care.
Greed: A fee-for-service model can prioritize financial gain over patient outcomes.	**Align incentives**: Ensure compensation models support quality care over quantity of services.

2. *Defense mechanisms*: Psychological protection of the ever-important self-concept from competing constructs and intimidating desires. Defense mechanisms are counterproductive in complex patient management. Recognizing when they occur and adjusting puts you back on task. Practical steps for improvement include:

> *Promote open dialogue*: Encourage team members to share their perspectives without fear of retribution.
>
> *Acknowledge and address ego*: Be aware of and manage personal ego to facilitate better team collaboration.
>
> *Foster equal footing*: Ensure all team members feel valued and empowered to contribute.

3. *Emotional intelligence*: The ability to recognize and manage your emotions and to recognize and appropriately respond to the emotions of others. Developing skills in emotional intelligence helps you check your ego when it is interfering with care collaboration. Understanding nonverbal cues and emotional states is critical for cohesive team dynamics.

Ground yourself; sit eye to eye and not bird's eye with your team. If it becomes about you and not the patient, you get in the way. Check your ego at the door and get out of your own way!

9 Essentials Case Study—Essential 3

Darla-Kay loved caring for patients. She worked as a nursing aid for more than 30 years, starting part time at age 16 and full time following high school. From a young age she found great satisfaction in improving lives most in need. Most of her career was spent in the hospital and nursing home up until about 5 years ago, when she made the leap to home care. She found it very rewarding, taking care of patients in their most vulnerable state—their homes. Unfortunately, she found this feeling less and less at the end of a workday. The pandemic changed everything. Nursing homes saw the worst outcomes from COVID-19. Staffing shortages in extended care facilities led to lapses in care. Patients were isolated from loved ones, even at end of life. Families became more assertive for patient advocacy. They also wanted loved ones cared for at home. Custodial needs, previously cared for in a facility, now placed on home care staff. The work became more physically taxing.

Just as Darla-Kay approached Mr. Rodriguez's front porch, Marie pulled into the driveway. It was like the air was let out of Darla-Kay's sail. Up until this point, she looked forward to her visit with Mr. Rodriguez, who while challenging because of his needs and obstinate behavior, she felt her visits made a difference. But things were so much harder when Marie's was around.

Marie hurried from the car to meet up with Darla-Kay, "Oh I'm glad I got here when you did. I want to talk to you about Dad." Marie's stress was written all over her face. Darla-Kay was aware of Marie's situation—sandwiched between caregiving for both her younger and older generation. Darla-Kay's empathy for Marie evaporated some time ago. Mr. Rodriguez's care exceeded what home care provides, yet Marie insisted on more. She most often accused Darla-Kay and other caregivers of providing inadequate care despite their increasing effort. This infuriated Darla-Kay, and she suspected Marie's desire to talk now would render another complaint.

Identify each element of ego at play.
What threats to the cardinal truth exist in the case study?
How would you mitigate these threats to the cardinal truth?

Feedback: 9 Essentials Case Study—Essential 3

Identify each element of ego at play.

Ego (Freud) or schemas (Kelly) are one's perception of the outside world. The care team (e.g., Darla-Kay) identifies quality of life as absence of disease burden and hospitalization. The patient's family (e.g., Marie) perceives quality of life as a dignified living environment surrounded by loved ones.

What threats to the cardinal truth exist in the case study?

Ego: Darla-Kay's self-concept (her approach to treatment) is threatened, so defense mechanisms (avoidance, i.e., withdrawal of care) have kicked in and altruism gives way to power assertion over the patient and family.

Burn-out: High acuity and high care giver involvement/dissatisfaction demand more time and resources of the care team. The team's focus moves away from benefiting the patient to reducing their own burden.

How would you mitigate these threats to the cardinal truth?

Listen and acknowledge the team's concerns. Provide supportive statements that highlight their successes. Ask, what would the patient outcome look like if we withdraw support? Remember the cardinal truth—health care providers want to help patients; helping them draw their own conclusions about patients' needs resets threats of ego and burn-out.

Reflection
Essential 3: Check Your Ego at the Door

- Do you dictate care? How can you empower others?

- The cardinal truth is the fact that health care providers enter the field to help others. How can you tap into the cardinal truth motivating your team?
- What defense mechanisms do you exhibit? Your team? How can you get beyond defense mechanisms for successful outcomes?
- How do you demonstrate to your team you are on equal footing and not looming above them?
- How is your ego perceived by others? Are you aware of your own nonverbal cues? Do you recognize and respond to nonverbal cues from your team?
- Take time during a meeting or retreat and go around the room, asking everyone to tell their story of why they entered the health care field. What did you learn about the team?

References

1. Freud, S. *Das Ich und das Es*. Vienna: Internationaler Psycho-analytischer Verlag, 1923.
2. Freud, A. *The Ego and the Mechanisms of Defense*. New York: International Universities Press, 1936.
3. Kelly, G. A. *The Psychology of Personal Constructs*. New York: Norton, 1955.
4. Salvoey, P., & Mayer, J. Emotional intelligence. *Imagination, Cognition, and Personality*, 1990: 185–211.
5. Goleman, D. *Emotional intelligence*. New York: Bantam Books, 1995.

CHAPTER 4

Essential 4: You Cannot Do It Alone

If you want to go fast, go alone. If you want to go far, go together.

This African proverb communicates a fundamental truth. Taking it a step further: The more complex the problem, the more distance is required and the more people needed. This especially holds true for complex patient care. Many programs see modest returns on interventions. The problem is they "go at it alone" or do not invest the personnel resources needed.

Ears before Edicts

In September 2021, I began transitioning to medical director. The organization had been without a permanent medical director for three years. They operated with one of their senior physicians as interim medical director working in tandem with the longtime CMO, together filling this role. The problem: both were retiring simultaneously. Given the large community need, this program grew from two to six centers across a large metropolitan area in a few short years. The CMO had been with the program almost since its inception, some 20 years, developing

DOI: 10.1201/9781003655084-5

long-term relationships and a reputation as a trusted, kind-hearted physician leader. In 2021, the COVID-19 pandemic was still a force, with capacity restrictions, confusing masking recommendations, staffing shortages, and global fear. All of this led to reduced services—lower capacity, meaning a smaller number of patients we could serve. Morale, quality of life, and cost of care suffered. Conflict between team members increased, team dynamics fragmented, and behaviors "unbecoming to the workplace" (disrespect, insubordination, absenteeism, "at-work absenteeism," and nonadherence to standards of practice) rose and permeated.

I didn't realize the stress and fear the team felt—pandemic fears coupled with performance stress, working with less staff and interventions available. Human behavior is universal whether in patient care or human resources. *Clinicians must understand managing teams is like managing patients; the rules are the same!* Just as health behaviors are a symptom of an underlying etiology, team dysfunction too is the effect, not the cause. If you treat symptoms without treating the cause, you will not achieve a cure. The team's dysfunction was a symptom of their fear and helpless feeling. It's akin to the check engine light in your car. If you see the problem as the light being on and intervene by disconnecting the wiring to the bulb, you will "fix" the identified issue. The light will go out, but how long will it be before you have trouble again? It's likely a bigger problem occurs because more damage has ensued. Unfortunately, I focused on managing surface-level problems—cutting the check engine light cord without identifying and managing the underlying problem.

I falsely believed what was needed was "strength." At the time I saw strength as decisive, enforcing, above those led, and certainly above emotional/behavioral workplace issues. While leadership has aspects of each, neither is all encompassing. Staffing shortages were met with directives—you will go where I say. Resistance (based on mental well-being and work–life balance/family needs) were dismissed. Workplace behaviors in violation of human resources protocols were addressed with consequences over curiosity for underlying etiology. Much like cutting the check engine light on a car, soon more problems with more severity arose. The real issue was fear—fear of growth, fear of work burden secondary to staffing shortages, fear of new leadership and direction, fear of the pandemic, one's internal fears of failure. Remember God gave us two ears but only one mouth because we need to listen twice as much as speak. I should have listened to the staff's concerns. I would have understood better and developed smarter solutions. *The essence of leadership is convincing others to voluntarily move from point A to point B. Sometimes those you lead may need to go to point C on their way from A to B.*

The Meaning of Life

If you remember one thing: *The meaning of life is connection with others.* Just think for a moment of a time or an event with real meaning in your life. You begin realizing that the heart of these moments involves your connection with others: childhood connected with your nuclear family, young adulthood friends and social circles (think back to college), marriage, birth of children—even professional accomplishments involve mentors and team members' support throughout the way. Employees find the greatest satisfaction in their relationships with their co-workers. It's no wonder social interaction at work outweighs compensation as a reason for employee turn-over three to one.[1] Military camaraderie kept me serving beyond my minimum commitment. Societal successes are collective successes, not individual ones. I will admit, as a lifelong introvert, this is a realization I came to later in life. Every person you pass is an opportunity. Because of our hectic schedules and deadlines, many times we forget and let it pass.

Strategic Considerations

While most of this book is geared for the front-line provider, let's talk a little strategy. Health care, not unlike any other business, has short-term targets. When managers focus on short-term goals, well-intentioned people become short-sighted: Go alone so you can go fast. We go from quarterly report to quarterly report, losing sight of the five-year strategic plan. Many high-risk patient programs struggle because only a few individuals at the top of the organization influence allocation of resources. Without front-line input, the C-suite cannot fully understand the problem, making it difficult in devising needed solutions. *When looking for solutions, include those doing the work; they are closest to the problem.* Involve front-line workers early in the planning stages. Giving professional health care workers latitude for changes empowers better outcomes. To use a football analogy, it's akin to the quarterback calling an audible. The coaches in charge instruct a particular play from the side-line. After the ball is snapped, the quarterback, whose line of sight is on the field of play, sees when the environment changes and is no longer advantageous for the original play call. In his expert opinion as a quarterback, he feels under these new conditions a different play is more advantageous. He calls an audible and changes from the coach's play to the one now needed on the field. *Allow your team to* "call an audible."

Leading a team is not an easy endeavor. You're probably wondering how a team leader is consistent with equal team members and relinquishing control. *Leadership is not synonymous with control.*

Leadership is motivating positive change through influencing others through shared understanding and values. In fact, leaders may not have a title or commanding role but nonetheless profoundly lead a group of people. A highly functioning interdisciplinary team can have more than one leader at a time, and leaders can change at various times or circumstances.

Organizational Climate and Culture

Successful leadership requires understanding and adaptation to an organization's climate and culture. It's important to differentiate the two. Culture is deep rooted. In health care organizations you find culture identification in mission statements or core values and usually include some version of high-quality care, positive health outcomes, and financial stewardship. Culture is at the heart of what an organization does and requires a foundational shift for change. For example, organizations committed to serving underserved communities require an organizational paradigm shift when moving away from underserved communities to caring for ones with more affluence. Organization climate is how people in the organization perceive and are committed to the organization's norms and beliefs. Climate is much more dynamic than culture; it's the place for leadership influence. Organizations with a directional culture require a climate where their people are motivated for movement in that direction. Organizational leaders must create a positive organizational climate for successful directional movement of followers. Successful outcomes require first an understanding of an organization's climate and opportunities for motivating others to the mission.

Building Your Team

Essential 3: Check Your Ego at the Door, level-setting your place and priorities, builds to *Essential 4: You Cannot Do It Alone* by ensuring your ego does not impede working with the team. In many ways they are hand in glove because this work is bigger than any one individual, and only the beautiful diversity of thought and ability among a variety of people breeds innovation and great heights. Let's start with composition of the team—varied skill sets with a seat at the table (see Table 4.1). Then we'll discuss creating a highly functioning team.

TABLE 4.1   The interprofessional team- key roles

Patient/care giver	Central to directing care based on what matters most to them. Care givers often provide key support
Medicine	Primary care physician or advanced practice provider providing medical expertise
Registered nurse	Skilled in triage and clinical interventions
Case manager	Navigator of longitudinal care, assessing clinical parameters, providing education on chronic disease management, adherence to the treatment plan, advocacy
Pharmacist	Expert in pharmaceuticals
Physical/ occupational therapy	Expert in rehabilitation modalities including manual manipulation, exercise, and electromagnetic therapies
Behavioral health	Conducts social, cognitive, and psychiatric assessments; coordinates interventions linking community resources; provides counseling and medicine coordination
Registered dietician	Expert in food and nutrition for health promotion and chronic disease management
Speech language pathologist	Expert in managing speech and swallowing disorders
Recreational care therapist	Expert in recreation-based medical treatment to increase patients' physical, social, and psychological well-being
Spiritual care	Expert in addressing spiritual needs during medical illness, grief, or emotional well-being
Community health worker	Trusted community member who understands its nuances and connects patients with nonmedical resources for psychosocial barrier mitigation

(Continued)

TABLE 4.1 (Continued)

Front-line staff	Includes nursing aide, medical assistant, transportation associate, and administrative coordinator, who are often the first patient-facing staff
Palliative care	Provides advanced training in palliative modalities, comfort care, hospice eligibility, family meetings, and advanced care planning

Keystone

Imagine an arched bridge over a river held together by three large stones and mortar. On each shore side is one stone. The third stone connects them in the middle. Removing the middle stone supporting each side stone, not only would make the bridge impassable, but collapse on itself as the two side stones would cave into the water. The middle stone is the *keystone*, without which there is nothing. Patients and their social supports including caregivers are the IDT keystone. Solutions or paths (bridges over "troubled" waters) occur enlisting them. The converse is also true, without their help, no solution/ path occurs. Patients and their social supports (families/loved ones) are key team members. The patient is at the center with full autonomy driving guided care; empower them in this role. Social supports have a unique role because they can have large influence over the patient and often provide something different than the health care system. Long-term relationships garner high rapport, an asset when change is needed, such as moving to a higher level of care, housing, or cessation of driving. Loved ones are available on off hours supporting food, transportation, or ADL support, lack of which drives increased ED and hospital utilization. *When we're stuck, we enlist family and social support.*

Strengthening the Team

Once you've assembled the team, the process of fostering team performance begins. *Essential 1: No One Is Beyond Help* introduced concepts of carry burden, intellectual paralysis, and the resolute fallacy. *Essential 3: Check Your Ego at the Door* defined the concept of the cardinal truth in health care—health care workers want to help those they care for. *Essential 4* leverages these concepts, bringing the team together because *You Cannot Do It Alone.* You begin seeing how the *Essentials* build on one another.

Earlier I talked about a team-building exercise sharing each other's motivation for entering this field. Its power lies in the unifying cardinal truth reminding us of our shared purpose. Acknowledge threats to the cardinal truth as the elephant in the room—ever present and affecting your team. We've previously discussed ego's threat to the cardinal truth. Second only to ego, burn-out is an ever-present threat to the cardinal truth. *Burn-out results from overwhelming stress with poor coping, interfering with providing exceptional care.* Overworked providers become numb and detached, going through the motions, losing focus on care mission. Focus switches away from best needs of the patient to getting through the day, right-fighting (counterproductively proving oneself right) with co-workers, patients, families, or company procedures or policies. *Recognizing when burn-out occurs and refocusing back to a patient focus* rejuvenates the cardinal truth. *Remember to celebrate success with your team; never pass up an opportunity to compliment a job well done.* Carry burden with its repeated poor results fosters intellectual paralysis, threatening the cardinal truth. Patients, caregivers, and providers alike become cynical, losing hope and forward momentum when guilt arises from inability to see positive outcomes. Acknowledge their feelings and let them know many aspects of chronic care are outside of their control. It's okay when things don't go perfectly.

Do More with Less

In the real world, resources are scarce and personnel are costly. The reality is budgetary constraints have us working with less staff than we desire. Donald Rumsfeld, the late former US secretary of defense, once said: "You go to war with the army you have, not the army you might want or wish to have at a later time." As you see by now, I am partial to US military supporting examples. I realize Secretary Rumsfeld was a polarizing political figure, but I find this quote particularly powerful. The stakes are enormous. In defense of the American system of liberty, failure is not an option. The only option is defending with the resources available to you. There's a similarity with health care. It's not an accident it too uses military time. It needs similar precision. In health care, lives are on the line—failure is not an option. But for health care, how do you make do with what you have? You must innovate.

When I led a team in the Ambulatory Intensive Care Unit (AICU), we commonly encountered needs for which allocation of resources was not available. *Personnel is the most valuable resource.* Value is key in this definition. *Value is quality/cost.* High value occurs when this ratio is high—higher quality at a lower cost is high value. In the inverse, low quality and high cost equals low value. The issue we faced was the cost of an interprofessional—the case manager. Unfortunately, as often is the case, the system only looked at the high cost. They had a blind spot to the associated high-quality care, offsetting high cost and increasing value. We were saddled with not having enough case managers for the need. Our nursing leadership developed an ingenious path forward—*The Nursing Teamlet*—based on frequent nursing "touches". Patient touches can be nursing visits or phone check-ins with patients. They did not need to be long encounters to be high yield. While nursing touches help reinforce key aspects of self-management, more importantly, they are opportunities for patient check-ins. Patients with chronic diseases have exacerbations. Recognizing when patients get in trouble with course correction is vital. Nursing touches afforded intervention opportunities through direct nursing intervention or escalation of care.

The nursing teamlet, predicated on appropriate identification of patient acuity, inter-professional communication, and collaborative care, drove results. The AICU developed a simple acuity classification. Each patient was classified as a 1, 2, or 3. The numbers reflected their prescribed office visit follow-up. 1s were seen monthly, 2s every other month, and 3s every three months. 3s were most stable, 1s least, and 2s in-between. Higher acuities were assigned a dedicated case manager. Those with higher number designations, 3s for example, were assigned to the nursing teamlet with a prescribed frequency of a nurse phone check-in. Changes in stability led to changing stability scores and movement between the nursing teamlet and case management teams. This required interdisciplinary team consensus during a team meeting ensuring the correct risk and intervention prescribed for the patient.

Both teams were also supported by a community health worker (CHW), a member of their community with depth of knowledge of community resources. While CHWs may hold certifications in some states, they are not clinically trained, often at an education level less than college. Because CHWs are from the same community, patients often develop greater rapport with them and build trusting relationships. CHWs more often identify needs and barriers to social determinants of health (SDOH), bridging gaps between patients and the clinical team. Being from the community, CHWs connect patients to greater resources than what may be known to their clinical team. CHWs are high value due to their low cost and high-quality interventions. Additionally, some states are permitting billable encounters for CHW services, further increasing their worth.

Following nursing teamlet implementation we observed improvement in key quality indicators. Comparing AICU patients not assigned to case management before and after the nursing teamlet intervention, the group assigned nursing teamlet intervention demonstrated lower medical utilization of emergency room and hospital services, improved health status, and increased indicators of quality of life.

Managing Helplessness

Let's go back to Seligman's dog experiment. How do you teach the dog with learned helplessness that pushing over the divider barrier will stop the shock? How would you approach the dog cowering on the ground? What do you think would happen if you approached the dog hastily and pulled it over the barrier and stopped the shock? How would the dog respond to you while under stress? Would it resist your movement, or worse yet, would it bite out of fear or frustration? Most of us intuitively understand to approach with caution in this situation. Approaching in a nonthreatening manner, developing the dog's trust, and guiding his volitional movement gets to the goal without resistance. It's less intuitive that the same technique is needed with a team in intellectual paralysis (relationship building and motivation for forward movement).

The interdisciplinary team needs to know you care about their best interests. Seligman's dog is much more likely to move with you if he knows you are guiding him out of the shock and not toward more potential harm. Fear, helplessness, and trust are ubiquitous—in animals and people. Remember, a team paralyzed by difficulties managing high risk patients is concerned a different direction may make things worse. The way to break down this barrier is through relationship-building occurring through empathy, connection, and mutual trust.

Leadership starts with empathy. Empathy is seeing or feeling another person's experience. Empathy is different from sympathy. Sympathy is feeling bad for another's poor circumstances. Empathy creates a sense of equality, whereas sympathy acknowledges division. For empathy, you must understand the others' story. This *(empathy) begins with multiple sessions of active listening, without judgment or problem solving* (there's time for problem solving later). *Active listening* demonstrates they are heard. It requires being in the moment, free of distraction, demonstrating interest through verbal and non-verbal cues with *curiosity questions—questions inquiring for greater depth exhibiting value to the storyteller.*

Examples of Curiosity Questions

"Can you tell me more about ..."
"How does that make you feel or how are you managing through that?"
"What happened then?"

Empathy is demonstrated through authentic empathetic statements.

Examples of Authentic Empathetic Statements

"I can imagine how difficult it can be managing such a challenging patient."

"Most providers would feel frustrated with these circumstances."

Once the patient feels heard and validated, next move to connection through mutual understanding of shared experiences or feelings, strengthened through vulnerability.

Solidifying human connection (life's purpose) occurs through vulnerability. *Vulnerability involves putting yourself in a position at risk for physical or emotional harm.* Imagine your closest relationships. What strengthened them? You'll find it's your willingness to be vulnerable (asking to hang out, a marriage proposal, sharing deep fears or feelings, or an "I love you"). Don't confuse vulnerability with weakness. There's true strength in being vulnerable—taking a risk of harm. Open and share with your team. They will connect with you on a greater level when they see your strength facing risk, humanizing the leader, and setting the foundation for trust.

Mutual trust is required for team results. Trust your team that they are willing and capable of excelling and give them the latitude they need, without which they are not able to proceed as they know how. The cardinal truth is that all health care providers want to help patients, put faith in them. For Seligman's dog, the leader needs trust that the dog won't bite, and the dog needs trust that the leader will lead away from harm and for better. Your team needs to know you are knowledgeable on how to get there. Show them. Talk the talk and walk the walk. Speak professionally, demonstrating your expertise in your field. Describe past experiences and successes and how they relate to current circumstances. Speak respectfully to others, dress appropriately for the occasion, and be punctual—show up on time and keep meetings on time. Your team needs to know it's okay to try things and okay for them not to succeed. High risk patient management is a hard business, and the disease process will have inevitable exacerbations. Let your team know *the goal is not zero utilization; often with very ill individuals, the goal is less utilization than before with improvement in quality of life.* There is strength in numbers. As a professional, demonstrate your professionalism through understanding knowledge and collaboration beyond your organization. Pull in support of best practices, collaborating with national society members and publications, especially when your organization has a national chapter (American Geriatric Society, National PACE Association, the Institute for Healthcare Improvement, etc.).

Leadership is not forcing folks in a direction but rather showing them this direction is the way to go so that they move there themselves. *When a team member has intellectual paralysis, ask them what happens if we do nothing? If we do not help, then who will help? If we can't do something because of a barrier, what else can we do?* It is true that every health care provider has good intentions, but for some the intellectual paralysis is strong. The question is how much effort and resources you want to expend getting there. There comes a point where for some individuals a particular team is not a good fit. It is better for the team and the individual to adjust them out, even though it may not seem so at the time.

Help-Me

Cass Whiting is a 63-year-old female with diabetes mellitus and secondary chronic kidney disease with neuropathy, depression with co-morbid anxiety, gait disturbance requiring supportive devices with co-morbid vertigo, morbid obesity with liver steatosis, hypothyroidism, hypertension, heart failure with preserved ejection fraction (HFpEF), obstructive sleep apnea, and gout. Upon admission to the program, her diabetes was poorly controlled with secondary skin manifestations including hard-to-control candida and secondary bacterial infections. She was promptly treated with the appropriate courses of antifungals and antibiotics, but due to her lifestyle the infection cyclically recurred. Cass was nonadherent to a diabetic diet and not appropriately administering her prescribed insulin. Her nurse case manager was vigilant, instructing Ms. Whiting on hygiene promoting healing and prevention. Despite her efforts, Cass Whiting remained nonadherent. The RN case manager (RNCM) began experiencing the resolute fallacy—the belief that an individual is unwilling to change their behavior. The RNCM noted the patient's long-term live-in boyfriend of many years recently passed away. She described how their relationship was co-dependent. While Cass Whiting was capable of self-management, her boyfriend did almost everything for her, including insulin administration, ADLs, and hygiene. The RNCM judged: "the patient is lazy; she won't do anything for herself and relies on her boyfriend to do it all!" Obviously co-dependent relationships are more complex, and we cannot pass judgment without knowing all the details. What's striking, though, is that Cass Whiting was experiencing a significant recent loss. Even though she did not do it for herself while her boyfriend was living, having to do things on her own now reminded her that he was gone. The team helped the RNCM realize Cass Whiting was struggling with abnormal grief, and until this was dealt with, healing and adherence were not possible. Interventions such as engagement with behavioral health services and pastoral care were devised from the team meeting. The case of Cass Whiting is a great example of one discipline, in this instance case management, struggling with intellectual paralysis and gaining insight and management from the interdisciplinary team.

Chapter Summary/Key Takeaways

Working with others is paramount in high risk care. The roots of teamwork are inclusion and great leadership. Recognizing and acknowledging certain team obstacles helps you navigate through them:

- Value is quality/cost.
- Personnel is the most valuable resource.
- Ears before edicts—listen to your team before directing them.
- The purpose of life is connection with others.
- Front-line workers' input is needed at strategic levels with operational decision-making. Empower them with autonomy for innovative approaches and ability to call an "audible" on the field.
- You must have an interdisciplinary team of equals.
- Managing teams is like managing patients; the rules are the same.
- Burn-out results from overwhelming stress interfering with providing exceptional care. Overworked providers become numb and detached, going through the motions and losing focus on the care mission.
- Recognize when burn-out occurs, provide support, and refocus on patient needs.
- Empathy is seeing or feeling another person's experience. It begins with active listening.
- Active listening demonstrates being heard through body language and curiosity questions. Active listening is free of judgment or problem solving.
- Organization culture is at the heart of what an organization does and requires a foundation shift for change. An organization's culture

is represented by its mission statement or core values.

- Organization climate is how people in the organization perceive and are committed to the organization's norms and beliefs. It is the location for leadership influence and therefore requires thorough understanding for success.
- Leadership is ...
  - Understanding others with influence through commonality and shared values
  - *Not* synonymous with control
  - Motivating others' movement in an organization's culture direction, measured by the organization's climate starting with empathy, shared experience, and vulnerability.
- Remember to celebrate success with your team; never pass up an opportunity to compliment a job well done.
- Vulnerability is putting yourself in a position of emotional risk—strength, not weakness. Vulnerability is the great connector and foundation of mutual trust.
- The goal is not zero utilization. It's a process; the goal is better than before.
- Pull in support of best practices, collaborating with national society members and publications, especially when your organization has a national chapter.
- When the team is stuck, ask:
  - What would happen if we did nothing?
  - If not us, then who?
  - If we can't do something because of a barrier, what else can we do?
  - Have we empowered the patient? The care giver? (Keystone)
  - Is there an opportunity to engage family support? (Keystone)

9 Essentials Case Study—Essential 4

Marie, Mr. Rodriguez's daughter and primary care giver, in speaking with her sister Anna, said:

> Making matters worse, Sophie's overtime was cut back, and little Tommy needs new school clothes. I'm having to pick up some temp work to make ends meet. I don't want to burden you with this. I know you help as much as you can in your condition. I really didn't want to call you about this because I know you had chemo today and that always takes so much out of you. I just really need some support again with the case worker. We want to take him home again and you know Felipe is no help …
>
> Anna also feels guilty as she would like to do more but is physically limited by the breast cancer that ravages her body. It weighs on her, not much unlike her own mother, who succumbed to the same disease a decade earlier. Back then Anna was very involved with her mom's care along with Marie and her father. Mrs. Rodriguez was a very devout Catholic. For Mrs. Rodriguez, her faith instilled in her preservation of life.

The IDT team working with Marie is at an impasse as the de facto care giver, given that financial, medical, and alcohol dependency barriers in the family persist. How should the IDT approach?

Feedback: 9 Essentials Case Study—Essential 4

Keystone: When we're stuck, we enlist family and social support.

Commonly teams stop with Marie, under the assumption there are no other viable social support options. Develop a systematic approach deducing social support beginning with other family members.

Family:

- Marie has three children. We know one is college educated, one struggled in the workforce and lives at home (assumed potential financial hardships), and one is a single mother struggling financially. Are there opportunities for different types of support here?
- Anna is daughter of Mr. Rodriguez and Marie's sister and is undergoing active breast cancer treatment. While she is physically limited, are there forms of support she can provide?
- Felipe is son of Mr. Rodriguez and is Marie and Anna's brother. He has severe alcohol dependency with ensuing medical manifestations. He is estranged from his children, but what is their relationship with their grandfather and aunts? Could they be a source of support?
- Community: Religion was important in Mr. Rodriguez's late wife. Are there church connections and support services the family can tap into?

Leadership Case Study

You are the primary care physician in a dynamic value-based care model organization. You directly oversee several advanced practice providers (APPs). A patient files an internal complaint against one of the APPs, claiming inadequate care. You discussed the case with the APP and concluded they did not appropriately work up the condition for the following reasons: a gap in clinical knowledge, inadequate interpersonal communication, competing demands, and bias. The APP says the patient is a "chronic complainer" but also notes several operational deficiencies. You recommend further training for the APP as well as formal clinical oversight as part of an improvement plan. In the complaint, the patient requests a meeting with the physician, department chair, and CEO of the organization. The department chair comes to you notifying that her request will be honored and you are required to attend this meeting.

Identify opportunities for connection between individuals.

What can you conclude about this organization's climate? Culture?

Are members of the team empowered equally? Why or why not? Do elements of disenfranchising front-line staff exist? What are some leadership opportunities?

The APP has multiple process complaints (why do we do things a certain way) What is going on? How would you refocus them?

Identify opportunities for:

Empathy
Active listening
Shared experience
Are there elements of burnout?
Identify opportunities for vulnerability.

Feedback: Leadership Case Study

Identify opportunities for connection between individuals.

Improved communication with connection between the physician, APP, and patient, in addition to between APP, physician, department chair, and CEO, reducing dissatisfaction and improving outcomes.

What can you conclude about this organization's climate? Culture?

The organizational culture values patient and family satisfaction and quality care, evidenced by their due diligence in responding to the patient's family members' concerns and requests. The organizational climate is one of disconnect between levels within the organization. Trust has broken down between front-line providers who do not believe upper-level management policy makers execute the organization per needs. Upper management does not trust front-line providers managing this patient's concern evidenced by their physical presence oversight in the family meeting. **Are members of the team empowered equally? Why or why not? Do elements of disenfranchising front-line staff exist? What are some leadership opportunities?**

Team members are not empowered equally. The department chair and CEO agreeing to oversee the patient meeting demonstrates a climate that front-line staff input into managing patient concerns is less valued, sending a message of mistrust to the front-line providers. The leadership opportunity, aligning with the organization's culture of quality care and satisfaction, communicates confidence in the front-line staff's ability in course correction with the patient. This message also reverberates confidence in the front-line providers' ability for managing the situation. The department chair and CEO should remain curious—what does the front-line staff need? What are barriers to success? How can management support and mitigate barriers? Opportunities exist for the CEO and department chair for continually checking back in on patient satisfaction and recalibration with the team along the way.

The APP has multiple process complaints: "Why do we do things a certain way? What is going on?" How should you refocus them?

Remain curious, looking for a pattern to the concerns that can be addressed, and always looking for the underlying root cause of the dissatisfaction. Connecting back to what is important to the APP builds rapport and a starting point in direction guidance. Refocusing back to the care of the patient will find common ground via the cardinal truth.

Identify opportunities for:

Empathy: Identify with each perspective: patient, family, APP, PCP, department chair, CEO.

Active listening: Focused attention with both verbal and nonverbal cues as everyone describes their perspective and needs with echoing back what was heard and how everyone can contribute to the others' needs.

Shared experience: Finding common ground—all parties desire quality care and satisfaction. Start there, finding common paths to the same goal.

Are there elements of burnout?

The APP demonstrates elements of burn-out with missed opportunities for patient communication with competing demands labeling the patient as a chronic complainer. The APP's multiple complaints on multiple processes are a symptom of burn-out and if not addressed, similar and worsening problems will arise like an engine with its check engine light on.

Identify opportunities for vulnerability.

APP: Acknowledge there were missed opportunities, asking patient permission to make it right.

Physician: Acknowledge opportunities for more oversight, collaboration, and openness—available for clinical questions/decision making when needed by the APP.

Department chair/CEO: Acknowledge their own fears of repercussions to themselves and the organization. Acknowledge missed opportunities of support for those they lead, patients, and families.

Reflection

Essential 4: You Cannot Do It Alone

- Who is on your team? Who should be on your team?
- Is your office set-up for conducive input from all team members, especially front-line staff? How can you make communication more inclusive?
- How are you connecting with your team? Do you exhibit empathy? How? Do you exhibit vulnerability? How?
- Do you acknowledge successes? How? What are some ways you can make this routine? How often do you express gratitude? How often should you?

Reference

1. Griffeth, R. W., & Hom, P. H. A Meta-Analysis of Antecedents and Correlates of Employee Turnover. *Journal of Management*. 26; 2000: 436–488.

PART II
INTERPERSONAL CARE

CHAPTER 5

Essential 5: I Care

I'm standing outside Kit Kline's exam room door, about to enter. In recap: Kit Kline is a patient in a bad place. She is our most frequent utilizer, in the ED several times a week for somatic and behavioral symptoms. Care givers and staff are burned out. Ms. Kline has a history of constant negative communication including both verbal and physical threats. Because of this, the police are notified when she is on site. Kit declined signing a behavioral contract, the court denied a guardianship request, and pandemic restrictions forbid staff's efforts for involuntary disenrollment from the program. I opened the door and went in.

Kit Kline was known by most employees because of her circumstances. I never met her in person. She was not at all what I expected. In the corner of the room, she sat hunched over her cane, head down, in the visitor seat with her left leg fully extended. She appeared debilitated and older than her age. I expected a more robust individual, given the police escort. It became quickly apparent she was not a threat. I called her by her formal name (Ms. Kline), introduced myself, and immediately sat on the doctor stool. Normally I would apologize for any delay, but since I came immediately to see her (this was my second scheduled

DOI:10.1201/9781003655084-7

meeting with her; the first she left before being seen because of a few minutes' wait).

I said: "How are you doing today?"

"Miserable, I am in so much pain. I'm tired living like this."

"I'm sorry to hear that. I've reviewed your chart; you've had quite a time of it. Anyone who's gone through what you've gone through would feel this way. I'm here to help you and get you feeling better."

"I don't know if you can."

"Kit, I know you've been through a lot, but give me a chance in seeing from a fresh new perspective. Is that an Army PT jacket?" I pointed to her Army issue jacket.

"Yes, my brother gave it to me."

"I recognize it because I'm in the Army, it's the older version. Is your brother in the Army?"

"Yes, he's stationed down south," she said.

"How long has he been in the Army?"

"He made a 20-year career of it."

"Did he have to travel much?"

"Oh yes, he never was stationed overseas, but he moved around the United States a lot."

"That's hard on a person and families. I deployed twice overseas away from my family. I know how difficult that can be. Those who serve sacrifice so much. Thank him for his service to our country. It's so nice he gives you his retired fitness attire. It's a nice jacket." I said.

"Thank you, yes, it is, I am lucky he gives them to me. He always gives me stuff like this." Kit Kline said.

"I understand you've been having a lot of difficulty with back pain. Come have a seat on the exam table and let me examine your back."

Kit Kline's exam was benign, only remarkable for lower lumbar para-spinal tightness with spasm.

"Kit, your back is in spasm; no wonder you're in a lot of pain. I'd recommend you work with our physical therapist, who can help relieve the tension and better balance your muscles, helping with the pain. Can I walk you down there now and let them know what I'd like them to do?"

Kit Kline was agreeable. We walked together out of the exam room, through the clinic, past the nursing station, and into the health center, finally arriving in the physical therapy suite. Along the way, we passed many staff members observing me walking side by side with Kit Kline. When we reached physical therapy, the therapists were finishing up their lunch. I introduced Kit Kline (though she needed no introduction) and explained my assessment and recommendations. They said they would be happy to see her after lunch and asked if Ms. Kline would like to have lunch in the health center while she waited. She agreed, and the physical therapist escorted her into the other room for lunch, following which she completed her physical therapy session.

Kit Kline continued having crises, reaching out to staff. Each time I had her come to the clinic and see me. Each visit began with some small talk, active listening to her concerns without judgment, and acknowledgement of feelings. Kit Kline expressed she was very frustrated with her pain specialist. Her implantable pain pump remained in place, but its medication changed from a narcotic to an anesthetic. Despite frequent visits with dose adjustment, the pain was unchanged. Like many others working with Kit Kline, the pain specialist also became frustrated. Their visits got shorter and shorter and often contentious. Kit Kline could not understand why he could not explain lack of pain relief. At this point I simply said: "Because he cannot get rid of your pain. As a pain specialist that is probably hard for him to admit. The reason he cannot relieve your pain with the pain pump medication is because your pain is now chronic and no longer elicited from your back. After years of stimulus from your back, your brain got stuck in a continuous loop. The brain now continually interprets back pain, even in the absence of a back stimulus. Unfortunately, it's worse with stress, emotions, and a poor mood. Acute pain treatment modalities work on peripheral pain receptors, not central chronic pain loops." This was a pivotal point. Kit Kline finally got an answer to her question. A physician took time and explained a hard truth authentically. For the first time she understood why the treatment was not providing relief. I went on to tell her that chronic pain is just that—chronic. It is never cured; it's managed. I could help her feel better, with tolerable and improving function. Life could be better. It was a turning point in her thinking: Her pain was not acute pain, and treatment for acute pain would not work. She began having hope that another treatment would. I connected with Kit Kline, developing trust, and later prescribed her an antidepressant. Because of our rapport, she took the medication (she was previously nonadherent to similar medications prescribed by other providers). Her mood began improving and so too did her perceptions of pain.

The most important element in prescribed health behavior change is provider–patient rapport. Rapport is defined as a harmonious relationship between individuals or groups with mutual understanding and bidirectional communication, acknowledging both parties experience a range of emotions in high-stakes encounters, like my anticipation of meeting Ms. Kline. These emotions may include anger, frustration, fear, avoidance, or sadness. It's just as important acknowledging and addressing these emotions in interprofessional teams as it is with patients. *Acknowledging and addressing anticipatory emotions both in your interprofessional team and patient/social supports is crucial for effective communication and rapport building.* Building rapport begins with empathy. Remember, empathy is seeing or feeling another person's experience. But how is this demonstrated to a patient?

Connecting with Patient Emotions

During residency I worked under Dr. Robert C. Smith at Michigan State University. He and colleagues developed the NURS(E) framework,[1] assisting providers in managing emotions (Figure 5.1).

NURSE employs when patients express an emotion. The practitioner must recognize both verbal and nonverbal (body language) emotional cues. Some examples include those in Table 5.1.

Once you've recognized the emotion, then NURSE it. First, name it. It's nice that in the acronym is the first step, but it's no accident either. It is the first because without this step you cannot proceed with rapport building. Naming the emotion does two things. First, it

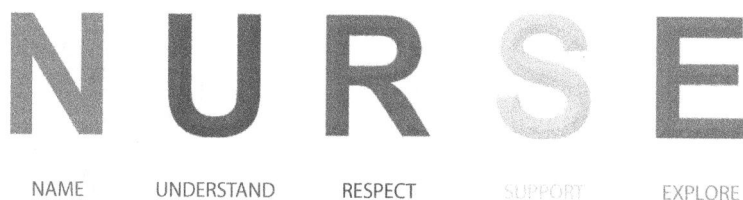

N U R S E

| NAME | UNDERSTAND | RESPECT | SUPPORT | EXPLORE |

FIGURE 5.1 The NURSE Acronym for Responding to Patient Emotions with Empathy.

TABLE 5.1 Emotional Cues

Verbal	Nonverbal
Anger/yelling	Withdrawn
Crying	Poor or no eye contact
"I feel hopeless, sad, angry, confused, frustrated, overwhelmed ..."	Slumping posture
Short or yes-or-no answers	Crossed arms
Distracted or tangential answers	Multiple somatic complaints
Describes an emotion or feeling	Fidgety, pressured speech, agitated

brings awareness to the emotion. Second, it establishes a connection with the patient, letting them know you are aware of the emotion and not afraid to talk about it. Patients are not always aware why they feel the way they do. It's powerful when a health care provider leads someone to their own understanding of how they are feeling. Naming an emotion gives it the recognition it deserves. Don't miss opportunities for naming a patient's emotion. Sometimes defense mechanisms may make awareness of an emotion anxiety ridden, and an indirect approach is needed. You can do this by suggesting the emotion as a possibility (Figure 5.2).

Remembering to *Check Your Ego at the Door*, acknowledging the possibility you may not always get it right (especially if you are a novice at identifying emotions). Understanding shows the patient "you get it!"

Show the emotion some *respect*. Emotions are a normal, healthy response to our internal and external environment. People are afraid of sharing them, see them as a character flaw or sign of weakness, and often feel guilty that they have them. However, will they get better if they avoid dealing with the emotion? Respecting the emotion gives it the recognition it deserves as an integral part of the patient's life, a force to reckon with, and shows that you as the provider get it and are ready to tackle it. *Most care givers do the best they can; it may not be perfect, but in most circumstances, they are giving good care—call them out for it!*

Let them know you are there to help them. Their situation is complex, and their experience has likely led them to *learned helplessness*. They are feeling no way out and isolated from help. Advances in modern medicine allow living more years with chronic disease; however, the health care system has not adapted and is still set up for managing younger, healthier people. A 20-minute check-up with the doctor is not

Naming
- This sounds like you feel sad.
- It appears you are frustrated.
- Do you think you could be depressed?

Understand
- Thank you for sharing, this helps me understand what you are going through.
- I see how important this is to you.
- I can only imagine what that is like
- Anyone in your situation would likely feel this way.

Respect
- Thank you for sharing (the emotion) I know this was not easy for you.
- I admire your strength in dealing with this.
- I realize how challenging it is caring for your loved one and despite these challenges they are getting such great care!

Support
- I'm here to help.
- I believe this (resources, discipline/specialty) will make a difference.
- I can help make things better.
- We'll get through this together.

Explore
- Tell me more.
- Help me understand why you think you feel this way?
- How is this affecting you?

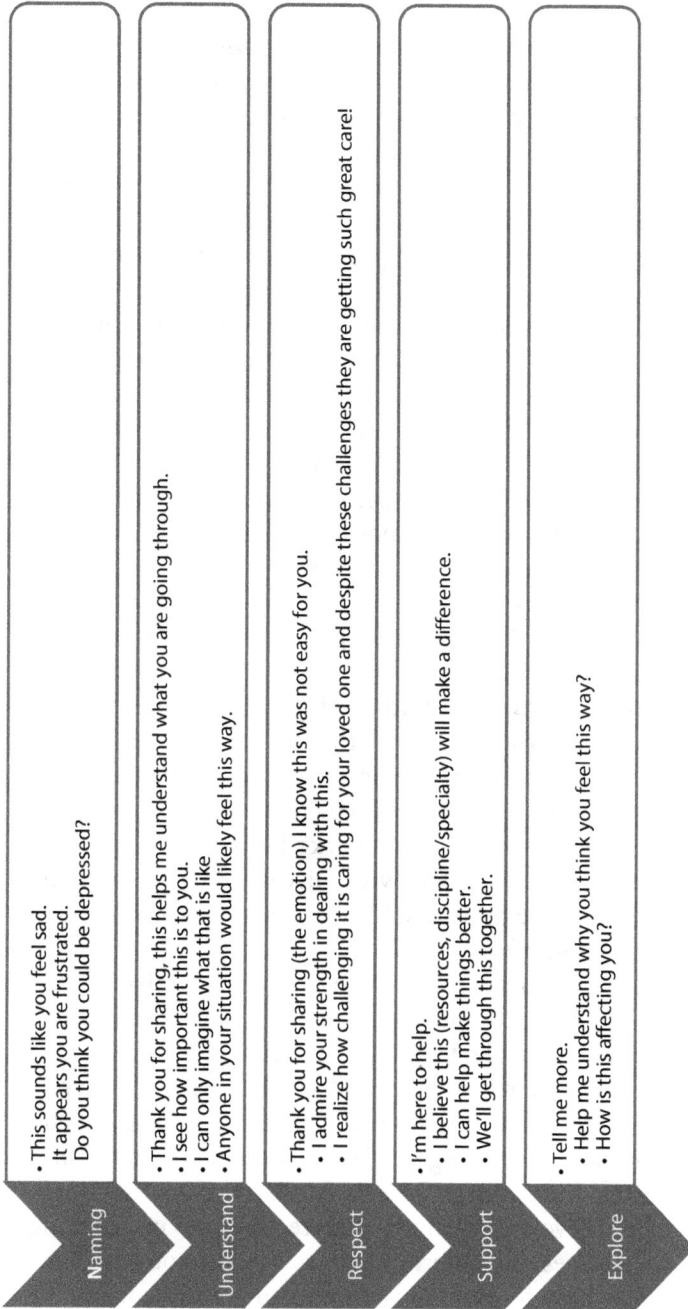

FIGURE 5.2 NURSE Statements.

enough for the chronically ill. Navigating a system of needs/delivery mismatch creates *navigation fatigue: Emotions and behavioral responses stemming from systemic barriers fragmenting care.* Patients and families become frustrated their needs are not met. "I care and can help" is often just what the doctor ordered. Once you've named, respected, understood, and supported the emotion, explore deeper levels for better understanding of etiology and mitigating barriers.

Psychosocial medicine was a required rotation during my time as an MSU internal medicine resident. One of the exercises included "psychosocial rounds" on the medical ward with Dr. Smith. Each resident took turns entering the patient's room with the group and began speaking with the patient and eliciting an emotion. Once the emotion was identified, the resident used NURSE. Dr. Smith recognized providers' pre-perceived notions—managing emotions is time consuming. This exercise demonstrated the NURSE technique is not. The group would spend only a few minutes with each patient. As we became more experienced with the technique, he started to put time limits on the encounter, reinforcing his assertion that it can be done efficiently. The first time limit was 2 minutes. It worked. He then shortened it to 1 minute, again with success. At this point he turned to me and said, "Bob, let's have you complete NURSE in 30 seconds."

Have you ever heard the expression that the A students make the best scientists and researchers, whereas C students make the best teachers? The idea is that students with natural intellect (the A students) are best suited utilizing that intellect. Students who work at it for average performance understand assimilating information in a way that clicks with them. They develop methods and techniques in teaching themselves the material that are useful to others. They know how to explain with meaning and hence make great teachers. For those whose understanding comes naturally, they have a hard time explaining how they got there, like explaining to a child how to balance a bicycle. In medical school, one student's class notes became the best study guides. For his own learning he organized the material in a certain way that became a great tool for the rest of the class! This book is my "class notes." I am not naturally empathetic or emotionally intelligent. I had to work at it, and the 9 Essentials are lessons that work. In fact, I am mostly task oriented and a concrete thinker. For example, the staff used to ask if I wanted to order lunch with them. Having packed my own lunch for the day, it appeared redundant to order another lunch. I always declined the invitation. I missed the point. It was not the physical lunch. It was gathering and having lunch together (a great way to connect with the team). My black-and-white thinking dichotomized lunch into those who ordered out having lunch together and those who did not sitting out. It never occurred to me I could have just as well brought my brown bag lunch and had lunch with them together!

As a young physician, NURSE was a series of tasks to complete. When Dr. Smith asked me to complete in 30 seconds, I gladly accepted the challenge. What happened next lives in infamy. I quickly fished hard for the patient's emotional expression, then blurted out each NURSE statement one after the other. It was neither authentic nor humanistic. The expression and jaw dropping of each member of the group, especially Dr. Smith, was remarkable. Dr. Smith is the ultimate optimist and positive thinker, always showing through in our "debriefs" in the hall after each encounter. That day, outside this room, Dr. Smith tried to remain upbeat in his debrief to me: "You did it in 30 seconds, but Bob, it came across as cold!" Remember that caring for this population takes time—give it to them. This goes for any technique in this book.

Demonstrating Empathy

Do you know *when* you should demonstrate empathy? Expressing emotion is a cue for empathy. Table 5.2 outlines more empathy cues.

I bet the last statement in Table 5.2 raised some eyebrows! You mean to tell me I should empathize with a patient who wants to sue me? Yes! *Check Your Ego at the Door and lean into challenges. It's always about them, not you.* Imagine the pain a patient feels when they feel they are getting inadequate care. Most malpractice suits start because of a breakdown in provider–patient communication.

Once you've recognized the opportunity, next display empathy. Following are some authentic effective empathy statements (Table 5.3).

You've probably realized by now the key to effectiveness in rapport building is *authenticity—a person's actions align with their values.* Simply put, you mean what you say. Without authenticity we cannot connect. Empathy is feeling what they feel. If you are not feeling the same, the shared experience is not there for a connection. Faking empathy does not work. Patients see through it, diminishing trust and therapeutic alliance. It's like Dr. Smith's feedback to me after going through the motions of empathy without feeling—"it's cold."

TABLE 5.2　Recognizing When to Express Empathy

Cues for Empathy
It's so hard.
I'm giving up.
I'm in so much pain.
Someone didn't do X, Y, or Z.
I'm dis-enrolling from your program.
I'm suing you.

TABLE 5.3 Demonstrating Empathy

Empathy Statements

I can only imagine how that must feel.

If I were in your situation, I can see how I would feel that way.

Most people who have gone through what you have gone through would feel like you do.

I can see why that's difficult.

That sounds frightening.

I would have also been... (disappointed, upset, sad, etc.).

I think you're right/I agree.

No wonder you're upset.

Active listening shows interest. Patients feel heard, which in and of itself is therapeutic. Active listening builds rapport. Use the LESS acronym in helping body language express authentic active listening: Lift-up: Sit with an open, upbeat, welcoming position. Make Eye contact. From antiquity, the eyes are described as "the windows to the soul." Look in and connect to your patient's soul. Sit forward, leaning toward your patient, not only is a symbolic gesture of "leaning into the conversation" but also to physically bring you closer to developing a deeper connection. Silence—listen more than talk. Remember you were given two ears but only one mouth; could it be talking is only half as important as listening? Use silence as an opportunity for them (not you) to speak again (Figure 5.3).

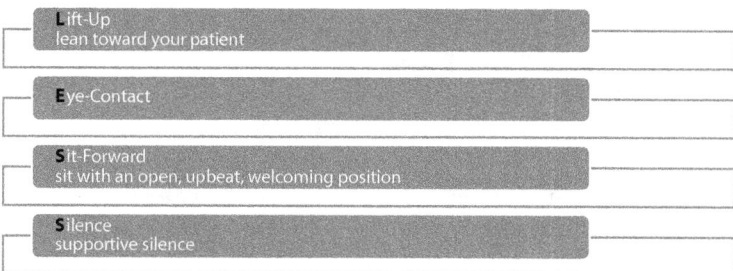

FIGURE 5.3 The LESS Acronym of Affective Body Language

Find common ground. We gravitate to those most like us with shared experiences and values. We are most comfortable in social situations where we relate with others. The trick is finding common ground. Most of the time, we can find shared experiences if we dig hard enough. Engage in nonclinical conversation around a book they are reading, an item of clothing, a common interest or hobby, or a similar shared experience. It's important to consider cultural sensitivity. Account for cultural context and individual preferences when responding to patients and families. *Cultural factors influence emotional expression and interpretation. Sensitivity to these differences is essential for effective communication.*

Culturally Aware Rapport Building

Today's modern world of travel, internet, social media, and multiculturalism necessitates rapport building through cultural competence—cultural awareness and sensitivity of cultural diversity. For health care providers, cultural competence involves navigating common cultural barriers (Table 5.4).

Most large health care systems provide some level of cultural competency training, and interprofessional teams should seek additional training if their system's training falls short. Effective programs include training on implicit bias, common cultural misunderstandings, and culturally respectful patient approaches.

Because effective communication is critical, language barriers present a very large threat to safety and outcomes. *A professional interpreter, interpreter services, or preferred language written material must be used in lieu of social support interpreters.* This eliminates potential outside bias in communication. Speak directly to the patient using the second person "you" instead of third person "they or them, he or she." The translator will translate verbatim, receiving

TABLE 5.4   Common Cultural Contributors to Health Care Barriers

Cultural Considerations	Mitigation Strategies
Health belief and practices (traditional, non-Western, or herbal practices)	Acknowledge their importance for the patient and incorporate them into the treatment plan when safe to do so.
Medical profession beliefs (mistrust)	Acknowledge and build rapport. Employ team members with similar cultural background as the population served. Community health workers are well suited in this role as they can often live in the same neighborhoods with similar education levels, which helps break down communication barriers.
Gender	Accommodations for same-gender providers as well as the use of same-gender chaperones.
Nonverbal and other cues	Cultural competency training for better understanding of cultural norms such as eye contact (respect vs confrontational) and punctuality (waiting times interpreted as lack of respect).
Faith	Acknowledge and demonstrate respect for beliefs. Leverage community religious leaders supporting patients.
Mental health beliefs	Understand and support patients concerned with stigma. Provide education on the science and benefits to mental health treatment.
Family values	Understanding cultural context in decision-making when it comes to family involvement. Proactively involve the family in care planning when patient desires to do so.
Health care navigation and literacy	Understand nuances of the host nation's health care system may differ from their own. Dedicated resources and time may be needed for assisting patients with health care navigation. Health care literacy differs around the world, and interventions tailored to specific groups of patients are needed.

TABLE 5.5   Language Interpreter Services

Service Sector	Resource
Private sector	Language accesses services: ■ Health care systems ■ Health insurance carriers ■ Pharmaceutical companies
Devices and apps	Apps: ■ Google Translate (not med specific) ■ iTranslate (has a med section) ■ MediBabble ■ PocketRX (medicine instructions) Devices: Live translation, e.g., Translators in a Pocket
Online	■ LanguageLine Solutions ■ CyraCom ■ The Big Word ■ VITAC
Software	Canopy Apps STRATUS
Government	HHS, CMS (US) Local health departments—many employ bilingual community health workers

information as if you were communicating to the patient in your own native language. Health care systems legally must routinely provide translator services. Technology, including smart device apps, internet sites, and AI platforms, offers real-time language translation. Additionally, most electronic medical record systems offer written health education materials in most world languages. Table 5.5 provides resources for mitigating language barriers.

Faith in Community

In the early 2010s, I practiced hospital medicine in suburban Detroit serving a large Chaldean population. Chaldean origins derive from what is now modern-day Iraq. While most of Iraq and the Middle East practices Islam, Chaldeans are Christian, practicing Catholicism as part of the Chaldean Catholic Church in the United States. The largest Chaldean population in the United States is found in metropolitan Detroit.

Preservation of life is a fundamental belief in the Catholic Church. Hospital providers, including hospice and palliative care teams, struggled with end-of-life decision making with Chaldean families. In one situation it became so intense that a patient's son told a palliative care team member never to return to his father's hospital room and proclaimed, "No one bring up hospice again!' A precarious situation; what should we do? A nuanced approach was warranted. Unfortunately, cultural beliefs are sometimes viewed as barriers to care rather than support. Believing they are a barrier leads down a path of intellectual paralysis and the resolute fallacy (Chapter 1). Believing cultural norms and beliefs are support breeds healing opportunities.

Since we served a large Chaldean population, we began looking at faith-based community partners— respected religious leaders who could help with spiritual guidance with end-of-life decisions. We asked this patient's son who his priest was and if it would be okay to ask him to join us in family meetings. The patient's son really liked us proposing involving his spiritual leader, thus increasing our rapport. Because he trusted his priest, hearing "The church believes preserving life does not obligate undue suffering through extraordinary or futile efforts" opened his mind to other care modalities including greater acceptance of palliative measures.

Relationships Build with Time

Relationships develop over time. Think about a relationship after a first date versus several dates or after marriage. More time together increases connection. Complex medical patients require frequent follow-up visits for monitoring their chronic conditions. Use this opportunity, strengthening rapport and cultivating the relationship. Rapport leads to trust. When patients trust their provider, they more easily follow their advice. *A word of caution on patient discharge/dismissal—it erodes trust.* Many practices have patient discharge policies including for noncompliance. This is an archaic practice that should be eliminated. *Noncompliance is not the problem. It's a symptom of the problem.* Discharging a complex patient, likely with psychosocial barriers to compliance, fragments care with poorer outcomes. Patients must feel you are in it with them for the long haul, without which true rapport and trust is not possible.

Let's review salient points of Essential 5 in the case of Kit Kline (Table 5.6).

Walking side-by-side with Kit Kline and engaging conversation with other staff in her presence demonstrated care and respect. I met with Kit Kline frequently, every couple of weeks and sooner when she requested it. The rapport we gained allowed her acceptance of taking the antidepressant. Her outbursts began dissipating. She became more patient with others and began coming to the center and participating in activities. Her pain continued but was manageable. She remains debilitated with chronic conditions, but her mood, activity, and quality of life improved and her ED/hospital admission rate went to near zero.

TABLE 5.6 Building Rapport with Kit Kline

Dialogue	Rapport Building Components
"How are you doing today?" "Miserable, I am in so much pain. I'm tired living like this," Kit Kline said. "I'm sorry to hear that. I've reviewed your chart; you've had quite a time of it. Anyone who's gone through what you've gone through would feel this way. I'm here to help you and get you feeling better."	**Empathy cue**: Miserable … tired of living like this. **Empathy statement**: I'm sorry to hear that … Anyone who's gone through what you've gone through would feel this way. **Understanding**: You've had quite a time of it **Support**: I'm here to help you and get you feeling better. **Active listening**: Leaned in, eye contact, squared up. **Authenticity**: Both parties trust the sincerity of what the other feels and expresses.
"I understand you've been having a lot of difficulty with back pain. Come have a seat on the exam table and let me examine your back." Kit Kline's exam was benign, only remarkable for lower lumbar para-spinal tightness with spasm. "Kit, your back is in spasm; no wonder you're in a lot of pain. I'd recommend you work with our physical therapist, who can help relieve the tension and better balance your muscles, which will help with the pain. Can I walk you down there now and let them know what I'd like them to do?"	**Respect**: Kit, your back is in spasm; no wonder you're in a lot of pain. **Support**: I'd recommend you work with our physical therapist, who can help. **Explore**: Come have a seat on the exam table and let me examine your back.

(Continued)

TABLE 5.6 (Continued)

Dialogue	Rapport Building Components
"Is that an Army PT jacket?" I pointed to her Army issue jacket. "Yes, my brother gave it to me." "I recognize it because I'm in the Army, it's the older version. Is your brother in the Army?" "Yes, he's stationed down south," she said. "How long has he been in the Army?" "He made a 20-year career of it." "Did he have to travel much?" "Oh yes, he never was stationed overseas, but he moved around the United States a lot." "That's hard on a person and families. I deployed twice overseas away from my family. I know how difficult that can be. Those who serve sacrifice so much. Thank him for his service to the country.	**Shared experience**: Is that an Army PT jacket?" I pointed to her Army issue jacket. "Yes, my brother gave it to me." "I recognize it because I'm in the Army …" **Respect**: I know how difficult that can be. Those who serve sacrifice so much. Thank him for his service to the country. **Authenticity**: Both parties trust the sincerity or what the other feels and expresses.

Chapter Summary/Key Takeaways

1. Rapport is a harmonious relationship between individuals or groups with mutual understanding and bidirectional communication needed for influencing behavior change.
   a. It is vital for health behavior change and positive health outcomes.
   b. It requires authenticity—a person's actions align with their values.
   c. Acknowledging and addressing anticipatory emotions both in your interprofessional team and patient/social support is crucial.
2. Components for successful rapport building include:
   a. Active listening (LESS acronym): Lift-up (open and relaxed body position), Eye contact, Sit-up (lean into the conversation), and Silence (supportive silence)
   b. Recognize empathy cues
   c. Demonstrate empathy (authentic empathetic statements)
   d. NURSE emotions (Name, Understand, Respect, Support, and Explore)
   e. Find common ground (shared experiences)
   f. Frequent check-ins/follow-up
   g. Give patients and care givers recognition
3. Cultural factors influence emotional expression and interpretation. Sensitivity to these differences is essential for effective communication.
   a. *A professional interpreter, interpreter services, or preferred language written material must be used in lieu of social support interpreters.*
   b. For health care providers, cultural competence involves navigating common cultural barriers including language barriers, health beliefs and practices, beliefs about

the medical profession and medical professionals, health care navigation and literacy, gender roles, nonverbal communication, faith-based beliefs, mental health stigma, beliefs about time, and family values.

4. Discharging patients for nonadherence erodes trust and should be avoided. *Noncompliance is not the problem. It's a symptom of the problem.*

5. A common barrier to rapport building is distrust stemming from navigation fatigue: Emotions and behavioral responses stemming from systemic barriers fragmenting care.

6. Check your ego at the door and lean into challenges.

7. The goal is always care for the patient. It's always about them, not you.

9 Essentials Case Study—Essential 5

The interdisciplinary team (IDT) convenes for a family meeting with the Rodriguez family. For this meeting as it's been in past family meetings, Marie, the patient's eldest daughter, is the only one in attendance. Both Marie and the IDT are exhausted and frustrated, having had multiple meetings with no improvement. The stresses of caring for Mr. Rodriguez are weighing on each. The tension in the room is high when they sit down at the conference table and the door closes.

What type of emotions might you anticipate in a family meeting?

NURSE each of the following statements a family member from the case study may express. Describe demonstrating empathy techniques for each statement.

- "I'm at my wit's end. I don't know how much more I can take."

- "I know it would be better to place Dad in a nursing home, but I feel so guilty."
- "You're the professionals. We came to you; why can't you figure this out and keep him stable and out of the hospital?"
- "I'm afraid we're losing him."
- "It's easy for you to say to put him in a nursing home. He's not your dad!"

What cultural aspects of communication are considered with the Rodriguez family? How would you navigate cultural barriers?

Feedback: 9 Essentials Case Study—Essential 5

What type of emotions might you anticipate in a family meeting?

Sadness, anger, frustration, fear, avoidant, or withdrawn.

NURSE each of the following statements a family member from case study may express. Describe demonstrating empathy techniques for each statement.

See Table 5.7.

What cultural aspects of communication are considered with the Rodriguez family? How would you navigate cultural barriers?

Rodriguez's Hispanic heritage may present some unique care considerations. Hispanic family values include interconnected family members with respect for hierarchy. Decision making favors a collective approach over an individual one. Traditional elder hierarchies remain with age. The Rodriguez family may desire more involvement from multiple family members as well as defer decision making or preferences to their father as the respected senior elder head of the family.

TABLE 5.7 Example of Using the NURSE Acronym

	Name	Understand	Respect	Support	Explore
I'm at my wit's end. I don't know how much more I can take.	Families in similar situations often feel over-burdened. Do you think you feel over-burdened?	If I were in your situation, I would also feel over-burdened.	I know you are doing the best you can under the circumstances.	We'll work together to find the help you need.	What makes you feel over-burdened? How are you holding? What social support do you have?
I know it would be better to place Dad in a nursing home, but I feel so guilty.	I am hearing you say you carry guilt regarding nursing home placement.	I can imagine how hard it would be to put your dad in a nursing home and see how you might feel guilty.	I imagine it's difficult sharing these feelings. Thank you for opening- up to me.	I have resources to help, including support groups of people in similar situations who understand and can help provide perspective.	Tell me more: What aspects make you feel guilty most?
You're the professionals. We came to you; why can't you figure this out and keep him stable and out of the hospital?	I hear a sense of frustration. Are you feeling frustrated?	I can see why you would feel frustrated. If I were in your position, I would feel frustrated too.	I admire your candidness in expressing your concerns and feelings.	I agree what we have been doing is not working; let's together explore other intervention possibilities.	What other options do you think might help? What are some interventions you control that might help?

I'm afraid we're losing him.	I'm hearing *fear* that he will die.	Most people with a gravely ill loved one feel the same way.	That could not have been easy to share. Thank you for trusting me with your feelings.	There are palliative program resources that can support you and that I can refer you too.	Do you believe Dad is at end of life? What do you think Dad would like at the end of his life?
It's easy for you to say to put him in a nursing home. He's not your dad!	It sounds like you might feel *isolated* that others do not understand how you feel. Do you think you feel *isolated?*	If my dad were ill, I might feel the same way.	I can see you love your dad very much.	Let's explore options other than skilled nursing facilities.	What are your goals of care for your dad? How can remaining at home align with the goal of care?

Hispanic culture generally follows Catholic teaching. Beliefs about the sanctity of life may influence end-of-life decision-making. In the United States and many other areas of the world, Hispanic individuals experience group marginalization and individual discrimination in health care. This can erode trust in health care. Furthermore, language barriers and education access contribute to lower health literacy in this population.

Approach the Rodriguez family as culturally aware: Involving multiple family members in family meetings, incorporating trusted cultural/religious influencers in assisting navigating family hierarchy and end-of-life decision making, building trust, and providing appropriate levels of health education produces better outcomes.

Reference

1. Smith, R. C. *Smith's Patient-Centered Interviewing: An Evidence-Based Method*, 4th Edition. Philadelphia: Lippincott Williams & Wilkins, 2018.

CHAPTER 6

Essential 6: Meet 'em Where They Are (and Bring Them Along): What Matters Most?

M y first encounter with Kit Kline is a great example of Essential 6. I met her where she was—*in pain*—and literally (and figuratively) brought her with me. It was much more than ending at the intervention (physical therapy), but walking through the halls of the center demonstrated to Kit Kline what mattered most—*Essential 5: I Care*. For Essential 6, meet your patient where they're at, in mattering most to them, and bring them with you to better outcomes. *Practitioners are often frustrated when their interventions are not taken up by their patients, but often the prescribed interventions do not align with what matters most to the patient.*

Hierarchy of Needs

When the Institute for Health Care Improvement (IHI) described *Matters Most* as part of the 5Ms framework, they described it in terms of what matters most to the patient's health.[1] Essential 6 takes this further. Health care providers are biased, believing health is what is most important to an individual. Health is often not top of mind for most individuals, especially underserved populations. In 1943, psychologist Abraham Maslow described the hierarchy of needs as outlined in Figure 6.1.

Maslow described stepwise progression of human behavior beginning with the motivations for basic needs of food, water, and shelter, followed by safety and security. Only after basic needs are met can individuals progress to higher needs (socialization, self-worth, and self-actualization). Too often, medical professionals focus on motivations at higher levels of the hierarchy such as health promotion, patient education, etc. But many times, a patient's most basic

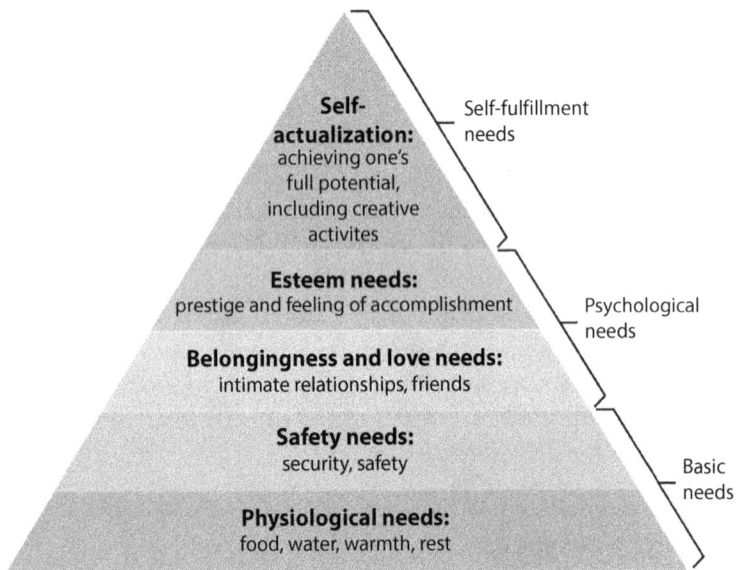

FIGURE 6.1 Maslow's Hierarchy of Needs.

needs such as housing or food insecurity are not met. Until basic needs are met, higher needs, like managing chronic disease, cannot be. Sometimes what matters most to a patient is where they are getting their next meal or where they are staying tonight.

Partnership

Once your team identifies what matters most to the patient, partnership begins. The interdisciplinary team must address any needs on the lower rungs of Maslow's hierarchy first. The art is marrying medical needs and interventions with what matters most to the patient. Take for instance a patient with congestive heart failure (CHF), with frequent exacerbations, who is nonadherent to a sodium restricted diet. The team may get frustrated because education on low sodium diet seemingly does not change behavior and results.

One of my pet peeves is the statements, "They're going to do what they want to do," "You're not going to change them," or "We can't do anything, they are non-compliant." They conflict with *Essential 5: I Care* because they are give-up statements. Because they reflect one-way thinking, they also erode *Essential 4: You Cannot Do It Alone*, because it side-steps interdisciplinary thought. The word *compliance* infers a hierarchical, top-down approach from provider to patient. The patient *complies* with the provider's recommendations. With compliance, most often, there is a mismatch in therapeutic buy-in. The provider more likely has more buy-in for the intervention than does the patient. *Adherence* confers behavior based on mutually agreed values. Compliance can get short-term gains but is not sustainable. Military structure is a good example. In short-term, life-and-death battlefield situations, compliance is needed. Even in the military, though, long-term strategy requires more than compliance for sustainment. *If you say a patient is "noncompliant," you've already lost the long game.*

Getting back to our patient with CHF, identify what matters most. For example, let's say its food choice based on taste. Assuming the patient understands certain choices increase their risk of adverse health outcomes, how can we partner in what matters most to them, for reducing CHF exacerbations? The answer could be adjustment of diuretics with focused intervention. The message he previously heard was to reduce sodium to 1,800 mg/day. This left him without the taste enjoyment that matters most. What if he could restrict or limit one high-sodium food? If he likes hot dogs, what if you could commit to having them less often (rather than cutting them out completely)? On the occasions when he has dietary indiscretions, he could take an additional as-needed diuretic dose. For accommodating a high salt diet, his daily maintenance diuretic dose could also adjust up. Realize this is not the ideal and carries increased risks. Remember the goal is *decreased, not zero*, exacerbations and hospitalizations. The patient is happier, you've met them where they are and partnered with mutual goals, bringing them with you on the start of the journey for better health outcomes. Rome wasn't built in a day, and neither is health behavior change. It's the beginning of the journey; the patient begins looking at their choices, cause and effect, with action (more diuretic with higher salt foods). It's empowerment fostering self-management. The patient may well change behavior and decline a certain food choice because it will require more medication and frequent urination.

Matters Most in Practice

I've seen teams struggle with what matters most for their patients. On the surface, it should seemingly be simple. It is telling when we struggle with patients we know well. When it seems we are at an impasse with a patient, consider the following:

- Go back to the treatment plan and conflicting patient adherence. What is getting in the way? What does the patient value, and is it in conflict with the treatment plan?
- Matters most can be matters most(s). Patients may have multiple important values; inquire until the picture is complete.
- When conflict exists between what matters most and medical intervention, it's helpful asking for patient expectations: "What would you like to see happen?" Understanding the patient's desired outcome helps clarify their values (matters most) and is a stepping-stone for collective partnership.
- Matters most can open goals-of-care conversations and help patients identify when conflict exists between the patient, family, and/or current interventions in place.

Jerry Madison's story illustrates the power of Essential 6. Jerry was a frequent utilizer of the ED. His ED visits were social, not medical, in nature. The team believed they stemmed from social isolation. They prescribed an intervention of increasing his day center attendance. This not only afforded an opportunity for socialization but also greater team observation. However, this intervention was unsuccessful: Mr. Madison would stay a couple hours in the center, then leave to go to the ED. This perplexed the interdisciplinary team. Why did their intervention not work? *When you get stuck, approach from a different perspective.* Jerry Madison's environment, both at home and in the program's day center, did not meet his needs, leaving him unfulfilled. The team then went back to the drawing board and asked: "What matters most to Jerry Madison?" Jerry Madison was a musician, and music mattered most for him. The team incorporated his music and performances into his day center routine. The result—no more ED visits! Imagine how the first outcome would be different if the team started from "What matters most?" Mr. Madison's example illustrates a fundamental principle—always find out what matters most before prescribing an intervention. Remember the "M": Never Make a Move before asking what Matter Most.

Returning to Wally Gustoff from the Essential 3 chapter enrolling in our program and anticipating spinal surgery for alleviation of his back pain. Unfortunately, following enrollment, he became sicker and more debilitated secondary to his multiple co-morbidities. His new network neurosurgeon and cardiologist deemed him too high risk for surgery. Wally became disillusioned. He blamed his new care team for keeping him from what he believed to be curative surgery. He stopped engaging and refused to come to the day program or clinic or to take calls from members of his interprofessional team. His CHF deteriorated secondary to poor adherence to sodium and fluid restrictions. He became volume overloaded, leading to more disability from decreasing functional ability. The more sedentary, the worse his back pain became. His worsening health status further curtailed his surgical hopes. His actions seemed counterproductive to his surgical goal.

Interestingly, the IDT identified that surgery or pain relief was not actually what mattered most to Wally Gustoff. What mattered most was rapport with his care team. He put his faith in his team for surgery and pain relief. He felt let down. He gave up, participating in self-destructive behaviors taking him further from his goal. Because he lost trust with the care team, he was unwilling to engage in their recommendations: "I mean, why should I trust you? You didn't come through for me." The team enlisted their members most skilled at relationship building utilizing principles of *Essential 5: I Care*. Only then could the process of working on managing pain, volume overload, and surgical expectations begin. *The goal is not perfection.* It's not an overnight process, is time intensive, and may never change the fact that Wally Gustoff is a poor surgical candidate. We may never change his thinking about curative surgery, but we can better control his pain, functional ability, number of hospitalizations, and quality of life.

Mr. Gustoff's example highlights the complexity of *Essential 6: Meet 'em Where They Are (and Bring Them Along): What Matters Most?* What matters most for patients and care givers is not always surface level. I have seen many teams report what matters most by repeating back what the patient says verbatim: "I want to feel good." "I want to live." "I don't want to go into a nursing home." Mr. Gustoff expressed wanting curative surgery; however, connection to his care team for health improvement mattered even more. Patients have deeper motivations. "I want to feel good" could indicate being free of pain or depression. "I want to live" could mean wanting to attend a granddaughter's wedding. "I don't want to go into a nursing home" may be a sign of financial concerns. For success, interventions must align with the appropriate patient goals. If finances are a barrier to a structured living environment, rather than remaining in their current living situation, the intervention is different. Attempts at maintaining the patient at home may be less effective than an affordable nursing facility. *What matters most is like an iceberg. There's more below the surface for the interdisciplinary team to uncover.*

Chapter Summary/Key Takeaways

Improving patient outcomes involves a partnership between the patient and the interprofessional health care provider rooted in shared goals. Establishing this partnership requires the interprofessional health care provider's understanding of what matters most for the patient and aligning the treatment plan with it. Meeting patients where they are is a process. It takes time and may not obtain the interprofessional's optimal results. Patients have autonomy, picking and choosing medical interventions to the degree they balance what matters most to them. Improving patient outcomes is just that—improving, not perfection.

- Remember "M": Never Make a Move before asking what Matter Most.
- Meet your patient where they're at, what is mattering most to them, connecting, and bringing them with you to better outcomes.
- Medical complexity often stems from poor care access secondary to social determinants of health. Evaluate basic needs such as food and shelter, addressing them first.
- Compliance strategy stems from one-way, top-down provider-over-patient goal setting. It is ineffective as a long-term strategy.
- Adherence occurs because of mutually agreed upon values and is key for long-term sustainment.
- Discussing what matters most to patients uncovers potential conflict between patient values and prescribed interventions. It can also often be a starting point for goals-of-care communication.
- What matters most can be multiple, cross multiple disciplines, and not always be apparent to the patient.
- Asking directly what matters most or what they'd like to see happen helps identify what matters most.
- What matters most is like an iceberg. There's more below the surface for the interdisciplinary team to uncover.

9 Essentials Case Study—Essential 6

Marie walks in scanning the room—familiar faces, the team caring for her father. As she is sitting but not quite seated yet, Katie, the nursing manager, begins, "I'm afraid we've come to a place we never want to be. Your dad's care needs exceed our capabilities. The level of care he requires for safety is facility level care." Marie starts to say something but is immediately shut down by Katie. "Marie, we have been over this multiple times, we're at an impasse. Your expectations are not realistic and are taking a toll on my staff. We have tried multiple interventions and staffing changes, exhausting all we can do. Unfortunately, at this point I cannot continue putting our agency in charge of your father's care. It's just not safe. If you're still not agreeable for placement for your dad, I'm afraid we're going to have to discharge him from our care. You will need to find another agency to care for him in his home," Katie said.

At this point, Marie's anger turned to sadness and fear. Her hostile outward appearance deflated. She burst into tears. "Oh no, you don't understand how terrible it is for Dad in a nursing home." Marie continues, "He hates it there. They neglect him, he's always wet. He constantly fights with them, and they just send him to the hospital to be rid of him. My father deserves better than this. I don't know what to do anymore, it's so hard. He can't come live with me. My house is full with two of my grown children living with me and dependent on me financially, not to mention my baby grandson. I don't know what to do if I don't have your help with him."

What matters most to the patient's family?
Identify elements of a compliance strategy.
Describe the disconnect between what matters most to family and the care team's goals. Identify opportunities for shared connection and how it can impact care and outcome.

Feedback: 9 Essentials Case Study—Essential 6

What matters most to the patient's family?

Remaining out of the nursing facility.

Identify elements of a compliance strategy.

"If you're still not agreeable for placement for your dad, I'm afraid we're going to have to discharge him from our care."

The family must comply with the prescribed intervention; otherwise, improvement is not possible, and it's take it or leave it.

Describe the disconnect between what matters most to the family and the care team's goals. Identify opportunities for shared connection and how it can impact care and outcome.

It's important to the family that the patient remains out of a skilled facility and in his home. The care team's goal is patient safety, identifying that the home environment is not structured enough to meet care needs. The care team has an opportunity to better understand reasons the family has for repeatedly bringing him home as well as opportunities supporting needs to common goals. The disconnect involves goals of care, where the care team is aggressively pursuing longevity (based upon a medical model), but the family is more concerned with comfort and dignity (remaining at home and out of a facility). Bridging the disconnect could involve an open dialogue on goals of care. A palliative approach, with or without end-of-life or hospice care, better meets the family's needs.

Reflection

Essential 6: Meet 'Em Where They Are: What Matters Most?

- What matters most to your patients, and how does it influence their health care decisions?

- How can you incorporate patients' values and priorities into their treatment plans?
- In what ways can you better assess and address patients' basic needs supporting their overall well-being?
- Are you focusing on compliance or adherence in your approach to patient care? How can you shift toward a more patient-centered, value-driven approach?
- What lessons can be learned from the case studies presented, and how can they inform your practice moving forward?

References

1. Age-Friendly Health Systems: *Guide to Using the 4Ms in the Care of Older Adults*. New York: Institute for Healthcare Improvement; 2020.
2. McLeod, S. (2025). Maslow's Hierarchy of Needs. https://www.simplypsychology.org/maslow.html

PART III

INTER-PROFESSIONAL CARE

CHAPTER 7

Essential 7: Cognitive Power

Mary Jordan is a 74-year-old female with type 2 diabetes mellitus, end-stage renal disease on hemodialysis three times a week, diabetic retinopathy, hypertension, and depression. She lives in the community in her own home with her adult grandson. She drives herself to dialysis and doctor's appointments. She does not follow through with specialty referrals and often misses primary care appointments or arrives late. When she does come to visits, she appears very put together, often wearing fancy hats and dressing to a tee. Her blood pressure is always elevated in the office. In terms of medication compliance, she reports, "I take them when I feel like it." Recently she skipped some dialysis sessions "because I didn't feel like it" landing her in the hospital. What are the next steps for intervention?

Unfortunately, Mrs. Jordan's health deteriorated over several years. She was labeled a "noncompliant patient" until a cognitive assessment identified moderate to severe cognitive impairment. Because she drove, spoke, and appeared very put together, a cognitive impairment was not suspected. Missing medication doses, dialysis sessions, and doctor's visits or being late to visits are all manifestations of her cognitive impairment. Cognitive impairment is the

DOI:10.1201/9781003655084-10

great masquerader. Patients develop compensatory mechanisms (especially in early stages), going to great lengths in concealing their deficits. For Mary Jordan, partnering with her live-in grandson proved an invaluable intervention. His assistance with medication management and transportation (to dialysis and clinical appointments) were key in reducing health burden, allowing her aging in place in her home in her community. She resisted some of her grandson's involvement, and her grandson did not always press her resistance. As a respectful grandson, he often struggled with role reversal as she previously was head of household and his caretaker as a child. Remember the goal is better, not perfection! (See Table 7.1).

As with most physiologic processes, cognitive function also declines with age. Physiologic age-related cognitive decline affects processing speed. Since IQ is left intact, we see many professionals performing well into their 70s and 80s. As with any physical deficit, we adapt and compensate. Pathologic

---

TABLE 7.1   Key Steps in a Cognitive Impairment Intervention

1. **Cognitive assessment**: Conduct a comprehensive cognitive evaluation using validated readily available screening tools.
2. **Partnering with caregivers**: Engaging Mary's grandson in her care plan for assistance with medication management and transportation to medical appointments.
3. **Medication management**: Utilizing alarmed automated pill dispensers and labeled medication organizers to aid compliance.
4. **Behavioral strategies**: Implement behavioral strategies for nonadherence and missed appointments, focusing on giving Mary control over small choices while ensuring adherence to essential treatments.
5. **Safety and autonomy**: Balance maintaining Mary's autonomy with ensuring her safety, particularly concerning driving and self-management of her health conditions.

cognitive decline and dementia syndromes occur with or without typical brain degeneration on imaging. It's progressive, affecting global functioning beyond executive functioning. Dementia is an umbrella term with various subtypes including Alzheimer's disease, vascular dementia, frontotemporal dementia, Lewy body dementia, and mixed dementia. Each may be associated with different pathologic mechanisms. Exact mechanisms are not fully understood, though tau proteins and neurofibrillary tangles are implicated.[1] A large challenge in providing good outcomes for older adults is the intersection of normal cognitive decline and early pathologic decline.

Differentiating normal versus pathologic mild cognitive impairment is challenging. *If you can't remember where you put the car keys, it's likely age-related cognitive changes. If you can't remember the car is in the garage, it may be something more.* Advanced and in-depth neurocognitive testing gives better projections on who might progress globally. Additionally, they help differentiate from other disorders affecting cognition such as mood disorders, anxiety disorders, and disorders of processing, concentration, or executive functioning. Always account for education level and prior cognitive function. Just as stigma exists with behavioral health disorders, so too, stigma exists with aging and cognitive disorders. We must also acknowledge discrimination and unfair employment practices play their part for many older adults. Many experiencing cognitive decline with loss of function worry about becoming a care or financial burden for loved ones. For these reasons denial and cover-up occur. Patients not only compensate, and sometimes overcompensate, changing the subject away from one they have poor memory around. Patients with mild cognitive impairment are very effective at covering up their cognitive deficits. They are the *great masquerader*. Too often well-intentioned medical professionals view nonadherence (with medications, clinic appointments, or other medical interventions) as acts of self-determination, when a cognitive decline is at play. *Reducing adverse health effects from the great masquerader requires universal cognitive screening in patients 65 and older.* Validated screening tools with high sensitivity, minimal administrator training, and ease of administration in an office setting are readily available at most clinical centers. Cognitive symptoms in clinical depression such as concentration deficits and cognitive slowing can mimic dementia, a phenomenon known as pseudodementia; a validated depression screening instrument should be co-administered with cognitive screening. More in-depth assessment is indicated when these tests do not match the clinical presentation or capacity are in question.

Once you've determined cognitive impairment is impeding the care plan, it's time for nesting countermeasures. Some of my pet peeves are statements such as, "He's going to do what he wants to do" or "You can't tell her what to do." The problem with these statements is they're a judgment. Each individual desires their own autonomy. People generally do not like others telling them what to do. My response is always: How is this person different from anyone else? Think about it, do you like others telling you what to do? This magnifies when experiencing loss of function (physical or mental) and loss of control in many aspects of their lives, i.e., bowel/bladder, activities out of the home, etc. The solution is giving them *perceived control* in most domains, *when the stakes are low and achieve care objectives*—i.e., what color shirt to wear today or whether they want to take their medicine with apple sauce or milk. Both choices give them some control and accomplish the caregivers' objections, namely, getting dressed and taking medication. *Unless there is a safety concern, patients with severe cognitive dysfunction should control most aspects of their lives.*

While memory deficits are very stressful, on occasion providers and care givers can leverage them for an improved outcome. When undesired behaviors in dementia occur (i.e., sun-downing), distraction techniques move them away from the behavior; after a few minutes they forget what they were distraught about in the first place! Examples of distraction techniques include looking through old photo albums, playing music or a program on television from their era or that they enjoy, even showing animal or nature images on electronic devices. In mild to moderate cases of cognitive impairment where patients can manage their medications with some assistance, I recommend automated alarmed pill dispensers reminding patients of medication timing, or blister packs or weekly pill containers with labeled days and times for administration. The latter are also visual memory cues in tracking medication administration. If a patient wonders if they already took a particular dose (morning, afternoon, or evening administration), they can simply check the med containers and see if the medication is there for the time in question. When medications are in a pill bottle, it's impossible to tell without accurate pill counts, which is not a feasible long-term strategy. To-do lists and daily calendars are helpful memory cues in mild cognitive impairment. Other successful management includes increasing social engagement and physical activity (Table 7.2).

TABLE 7.2   Understanding Cognitive Decline

Normal Aging

As people age, processing speed decreases while IQ remains intact, allowing many professionals to function well into their 70s and 80s.

Pathological Cognitive Decline

Conditions such as Alzheimer's disease, vascular dementia, and others involve progressive, global functional impairment. These can often be masked by the patient's compensatory mechanisms.

Identifying Cognitive Impairment

■ *Common signs*: Forgetfulness, missing appointments, medication nonadherence, and unexplained behavioral changes.

■ *Screening*: Routine cognitive screening for patients 65 and older helps identify impairments early.

Managing Cognitive Impairment

■ *Communication*: Avoid judgments and understand the patient's perspective. Use motivational interviewing to explore their values and preferences.

■ *Interdisciplinary approach*: Engage a team of health care providers, caregivers, and family members to create a comprehensive care plan.

■ *Behavioral management*: Use distraction techniques and leverage memory deficits to manage undesired behaviors.

■ *Medication adherence*: Implement practical tools like pill organizers and automated dispensers to support medication compliance.

Practical Tips for Caregivers

■ *Giving choices*: Allow patients to make decisions on low stakes matters to preserve their sense of control.

■ *Distraction techniques*: Use activities like looking through photo albums, listening to music, or engaging in simple household tasks to distract and calm agitated patients.

■ *Safety first*: Always prioritize safety while balancing the patient's need for autonomy.

Chapter Summary/Key Takeaways

■ Cognitive changes occur as a normal part of aging. Pathologic cognitive decline occurs with high frequency in the elderly.

■ Beware of the *great masquerader*—masking cognitive decline symptoms due to fear, stigma, denial, and compensation mimicking medical nonadherence.

- Screen all high risk patients or those age 65 and over for cognitive impairment at least annually.
- Pseudodementia—Depression symptoms can mimic dementia. Screen for depression with cognitive screening.
- Memory deficits can be advantageous. Employ distraction techniques (looking through old photo albums, playing music or a program on television from their era or they enjoy animal, or nature images on electronic devices, etc.). After a few minutes, a severely cognitively impaired individual will forget what was distressing them.
- Unless compromising safety, cognitively impaired individuals should have autonomy over most aspects of their lives. Choices give patients a perception of control when the stakes are low, and all choices accomplish care objectives.
- Use of medication organizers, including alarmed automated dispensers, increases compliance and reduces adverse effects in patients with cognitive impairment.
- To-do lists and daily calendars are helpful memory cues in mild cognitive impairment.
- Increasing social engagement and physical activity improve outcomes in patients with cognitive impairment.

Managing Behavioral Aggression

- **Patient partnership:** Engage patients in decision making and give them choices to reduce feelings of loss of control.
- **Non-intervention:** Only intervene if there is an immediate safety risk. Use distraction and re-engagement to de-escalate situations.
- **Meaningful activities:** Involve patients in activities they enjoy or find meaningful to reduce agitation and improve their sense of purpose.

9 Essentials Case Study—Essential 7

Remember Darla-Kay, the home nursing aide, struggling with managing Mr. Rodriguez's family expectations; she had more reasons why she did not like seeing Mr. Rodriguez with his daughter Marie. Marie's demeanor and approach with Mr. Rodriguez made him more agitated, unreasonable, not directable, with outbursts of agitation. Once Marie even got caught in the crossfire, being hit by Mr. Rodriguez flailing his arms during an outburst. She struggled with understanding why Marie could not see what was obvious to her. After many failed attempts at Mr. Rodriguez living independently, he's now a large, real safety concern. Darla-Kay feels the care team's efforts are futile and therefore should be suspended.

How would you counsel the family on managing the patient's behavioral aggression?

What are examples of occult cognitive impairment?

How can you improve medication adherence in cognitively impaired patients?

Feedback: 9 Essentials Case Study—Essential 7

How would you counsel the family on managing the patient's behavioral aggression?

Managing behavioral disturbances in dementia involves patient partnership. Give choices when possible, and only intervene if there is an immediate safety risk. Distract or re-engage when behaviors start escalating. Do not argue or disagree (unless attempting an action such as touching a hot stove). Moods will pass. Memory deficits allow aggressive feelings to be forgotten. Engage with activities the patient finds pleasurable such as music, TV, reminiscing with photo albums, crafts, physical activity, or household chores such as folding clothes. If an elderly woman worked in the home, give her something to do like drying dishes even if you need to wet them first. If an elderly man worked with his hands, enlist his help "fixing" something even if you need to dismantle it first. Patients with dementia, like anyone else, want to feel needed and helpful. With agitation sometimes they just need a low energy state—reduce stimuli such as TV or other distractions, even turning down the lights, may help settle them down.

What are examples of occult cognitive impairment?

Frequently changing the topic of conversation away from areas of deficit.

Giving excuses as to why something cannot happen such as a home visit, med container check, etc.

Nonadherence to prescribed regimen.

Missed, cancelled, or late appointments.

Recognizing Occult Cognitive Impairment

- **Conversation patterns:** Patients may change topics frequently or give excuses to avoid exposing their cognitive deficits.
- **Adherence issues:** Nonadherence to treatment plans and missed appointments can indicate cognitive impairment.

How can you improve medication adherence in cognitively impaired patients?

Improving Medication Adherence in Cognitive Impairment

- **Medication organizers:** Use pill containers, blister packs, and automated dispensers with alarms to help patients manage their medications.
- **Visual cues:** Employ to-do lists and daily calendars as memory aids to support adherence to treatment plans.

Reference

1. Grundke-Iqbal, I., & Iqbal, K. Abnormal Phosphorylation of the Microtubule-Associated Protein Tau (tau) in Alzheimer Cytoskeletal Pathology. *Proceedings of the National Academy of Sciences of the United States of America*. 1986; 83(13): 4913–4917.

CHAPTER 8

Essential 8: Gotta Move

In the latter part of my grandfather's life, he became a complex patient. He was part of the "greatest generation," growing up in the Great Depression and selflessly serving in World War II. He understood an honest day's work embodying a strong work ethic. He was working class, and unfortunately physical labor had a toll on his body, beginning with severe osteoarthritis of the knee necessitating an early retirement at age 57. Like so many of his generation, he smoked, but shortly after the Surgeon General's Report on Smoking and Health,[1] my grandfather quit—cold-turkey.

At age 69 he underwent a coronary artery bypass graft (CABG) for four-vessel coronary artery disease (CAD) following regular interaction with the health care system. By the time he reached age 87 his "problem list" included CAD, COPD, diastolic CHF, chronic atrial fibrillation on long-term anticoagulation, prediabetes, mild–moderate aortic stenosis, and anxiety. My grandmother was six years his senior and developed dementia. He became her primary care giver.

His functional ability, despite these challenges, remained good. Aside from an occasional hospitalization for a CHF or COPD exacerbation, his activity

DOI:10.1201/9781003655084-11

was not limited for a man his age. He walked with the same cane (which was mostly used as a "walking stick" instead of supporting his gait) he had since his early retirement at age 57. He was still independent and still driving until a mechanical fall left him with an intertrochanteric hip fracture. Because of his advanced age and co-morbidities, fixation with hardware (nailing) was chosen through spinal anesthesia over total hip arthroplasty with general anesthesia. This left altered anatomy with functional deficits. He was now reliant on a walker for mobility, never drove again, and lost the ability to live in his home of 50 years, moving into assisted living. This necessitated a physical separation from my grandmother, who was then placed in a dementia care facility. Unfortunately, my grandparents spent the rest of their days apart in facilities. I wonder how their quality of life would have been different if the fall could have been prevented. Would he have more independence? Could they have remained together in their long-time home?

Like many other areas of health care previously discussed, patient mobility and fall prevention is reactive, not proactive. Additionally, physical and occupational therapy (PT/OT) modalities are geared more to maintaining function rather than *improving* function. Reimbursement is tied to secondary rather than primary prevention. PT/OT and durable medical equipment (DME) become covered entities once an event such as a fall occurs. Physical and occupational therapy insurance authorization is for a finite number of sessions instead of tailored to a patient's need, which is often ongoing. Where is the need in justification for the cost of care? Again, let's change our thinking. What if insurance covered upstream management with reimbursement for preventative modalities including restorative therapy, home safety evaluations/interventions, and DME for the most at risk to reduce downstream health burden and costs?

Essential 8 needs Essential 2: the right care (primary prevention) in the right place (patient's home ahead of a fall rather than a subacute rehab facility following a fall) at the right time (before, not after, a fall).

Assessing Mobility

Move it or lose it. This phrase is on steroids with advanced age: The less activity and movement, the more deconditioning and loss of function magnifies with age. Loss of function and deterioration is quicker and more severe as we grow older, with longer rehab time and diminished recovery. In fact, *the Fountain of Youth is* (wait for it) *exercise and activity.* Falls resulting from diminished functional ability account for $50 billion a year in nonfatal medical costs and some $754 million annual medical expenditure for fatal falls,[2] with a rising incidence of falls increasing 1.5% annually.[3] A mechanical chance fall in a high-functioning older adult can devastate fragile intracranial vessels and osteoporotic bones. Table 8.1 is a quick and dirty fall assessment.

Other validated tolls are included in Table 8.2.

TABLE 8.1 Simple Fall Assessment

# of falls in the last year	0
	1
	2 or more
Feeling unsteady on your feet	Yes = 1
	No = 0
History of injury from fall	Yes = 1
	No = 0
Total	0 Low Risk
	1–2 Moderate Risk
	3+ High Risk

TABLE 8.2   Validated Fall Assessments

Test	Fall Risk
Timed up and go (TUG)	> 12 seconds = fall risk
30-second chair stand	≤ 14 stands = fall risk
Four-stage balance test	Cannot complete tandem stand for 10 seconds = fall risk

Don't Panic, Stay COMMSS

Reducing fall risk crosses all members of the inter-disciplinary team, and is every interprofessional team member's responsibility. Moving from moderate to high risk requires COMMSS. Again, my military background comes through. In the military "comms" is colloquial for communications, usually radio communication, but also includes telecommunications including internet and satellite. Modern warfare involves sophisticated technology: Aligning high-tech, precision modalities such as drone aircraft in a coordinated melody of timing and accuracy for mission success. We need military-type precision in improving functional ability for older and high-risk patients. Table 8.3 describes COMMSS.

TABLE 8.3   COMMSS

COMMSS	Assessment	Intervention
Cognitive	Assess cognitive function: Screen 65 and older annually	Enlist social support, care giver education: Slow, purposeful movements, skilled and ancillary services, cameras and bed alarms
Orthostatic blood pressure	Assess orthostatic vital signs	Medication adjustments, timed and measurable fluid administration

(Continued)

TABLE 8.3 (Continued)

COMMSS	Assessment	Intervention
Medical, **M**edicine, and **M**anhattans	Assess medical conditions, medications, and alcohol use	Specialty coordination, medication management, cholecalciferol (D3) 600–800 IUs up to 1,000 IUs, ETOH education and support
Mobility and **M**icturition	Physical therapy assessment. Assess mobility aids—need, appropriate use, and barriers to use. Assess for bowel and bladder issues including urgency and incontinence contributions to fall risk	Memory cues for DME: Briefs, bedside urinals and commodes, medication adjustment
Seeing and **S**ensing	Assess vision/ lighting and sensation barriers to ambulation including neuropathy and loss of proprioception (sense of where extremities are in space in time)	Increase ambient light especially at night, ophthalmology referral, medication management, occupational therapy
Shoes and (home) **S**afety	Assess footwear and home safety including clutter/throw rugs, pets, grab bars, low bed, need for helmets, mats, raised toilet seats	Appropriate footwear, podiatry as needed, home safety evaluation, pet education, medical alert system, patient and care giver education, DME supplies

Cognitive

Each Essential builds on one another. *Essential 8: Gotta Move* is supported by *Essential 7: Cognitive Power*. Nonadherence for mobility aid use, just as for medication use, can relate to diminished cognitive functioning. Cognitive testing may offer clues for intervention. Social support including care giver education are essential. Aging diminishes the body's compensatory mechanisms for equilibrium. The body's ability in regaining balance is impaired. Many older patients do not realize their ability for preventing a fall from a minor tip off balance is significantly diminished. Sudden changes in movement such as suddenly darting in a different direction when the phone rings will lead to a fall rather than recovery upright if they began going too far in that direction. Educate patients to always think about their next movement, move slowly in the desired direction (especially up from a sitting or lying position), and avoid sudden movements or change in direction.

Orthostatic Blood Pressure Changes

Orthostatic vital signs will often clue you in to the etiology of falls and should be done as part of a fall assessment with or without pre-syncopal symptoms. Decreased compensatory mechanisms including thirst in older and frail adults increases risk of symptomatic low blood pressure, with rising from lying or sitting contributing to falls.

Medical, Medicine, and Manhattans

- *Medical*: Assess for neurologic, metabolic bone absorption (osteopenia and osteoporosis), psychiatric, and cardiopulmonary conditions affecting functional ability.
- *Medications*
  - Medications increasing fall risk: Psychoactive medications, sedatives, anti-seizure medications, pain medications including narcotics and muscle relaxers, anti-glycemic agents, Parkinson's medications, and chemotherapeutic anti-neoplastic agents.
  - Medications increasing risk of fall injury: Steroids, anticoagulants, proton-pump inhibitors, estrogens, and psychoactive medications.

- *ETOH Use*: Screen for alcohol use.
- *Mobility aids*: Assess for need, appropriate use, and barriers to use. Provide equipment, education, and barrier mitigation as appropriate.
- *Micturition*: Assess for urgency incontinence with appropriate interventions for mitigation (medications, incontinence pads, etc.).

Seeing and Sensing

Visual acuity declines with age, starting around age 40 with presbyopia. Cataracts, diabetic retinopathy, and macular degeneration account for much of the visual disturbance in the elderly with staggering health care costs. It is therefore not surprising older adults fall often because they do not see well. Check vision, and if they have not seen the friendly neighborhood ophthalmologist in some time, send them in for an evaluation and management. Provide recommendations for ambient light especially during night hours. Assess and refer for management of sensory deprivation including neuropathy and loss of proprioception (sense of where extremities are in space in time) affecting mobility.

Shoes and (Home) Safety

Footwear: Physics dictates structure. Vertical strength is directly proportional to the strength of the foundation. The stronger the foundation, the stronger the vertical structure. Our feet are the foundation of our upright bodies. In general, most footwear is inadequate in support for several factors: We often choose shoes based on look over function (think of high heels), ease of use (slip-on, flip-flops), or expense: wearing shoes well beyond their expiration date. With so many complex older adults being "vertically challenged," a solid foundation of supportive footwear is paramount. Shoes should be supportive with distributive offloading of tensile forces, i.e., low-healed, rubber soled, non-skid footwear. Discard worn shoes because uneven wear creates uneven force vectors moving in an unbalanced direction, precipitating a fall. Likewise, worn shoes lose arch support, and just like a building with a bend in its I-beam, the supported structure will tumble and fall. Diabetic shoes provide great support with offloading and are covered by many insurances and Medicare. Shoes need a snug fit. Avoid laced shoes for obvious reasons.

Home safety evaluation identifies trip hazards such as clutter or throw rugs, as well as other supports needed such as grab handles, low beds, helmets, floor mats, raised toilet seats, or device-accessible bathrooms. Medical alert systems are commercially available and are lifesaving and should be considered in any patient at high fall risk.

Follow-Up

When falls occur, close follow-up is indicated, preferably within 30 days. It is important for assessing progress and risk reduction strategies including any barrier mitigation. Referral to a comprehensive fall prevention program should be considered when available. Key components of comprehensive fall prevention programs include patient education and transition to maintenance, low-impact exercise programs.

Chapter Summary/Key Takeaways

Healthy mobility is foundational for quality aging. The goal is maximizing function. Modalities include physical therapy rehabilitation and low-impact exercise.

1. Fall risk
   a. Number of falls
   b. Unsteady gait: TUG test, 30-second chair stand, four-stage balance test

c. Need for a mobility device
d. Injury

2. COMMSS: See Table 8.4.
3. Follow-Up

a. Close follow-up (30-day)
b. Patient education
c. Risk reduction with barrier mitigation
d. Transition to maintenance low-impact exercise program

TABLE 8.4 COMMS Summary

Cognitive	Cognitive Assessment
Orthostatic vital signs (VS)	Check orthostatic VS
Medical, Medicine, and Manhattans	Evaluate and manage neurologic, cardiopulmonary, bone health, medicines, and alcohol use
Mobility and Micturition	Assess mobility, mobility aid needs and use, and urgency/incontinence
Seeing and Sensing	Vision assessment and ophthalmology referral, occupational therapy assessment
Shoes and Safety	Assess feet and footwear; home safety evaluation and DME supports

Essential 8 Case Study

Joe Patterson is a 70-year-old man with Parkinson's disease, essential hypertension, and hypothyroidism. He recently moved in with his daughter due to recurrent falls while living alone. He sustained two vertebral compression fractures on two different falls. He presents as a new patient, accompanied by his daughter with the use of a walker. Since moving in with his daughter, his falls have decreased, but he had two significant falls in her home: One in the middle of

TABLE 8.5   COMMS Assessment for Joe Patterson

COMMSS	Findings
Cognitive	MoCA = 16/30; moderate cognitive impairment
Orthostatic vital signs (VS)	Orthostatic vital signs—negative
Medical, Medicine, and Manhattans	Parkinson's disease, diabetes mellitus, essential hypertension, and hypothyroidism
	Meds: Aspirin, levothyroxine, hydrochlorothiazide, Carbidopa/Levodopa
	No alcohol use
Mobility and Micturition	Shuffling gait; uses four-wheeled walker
	Urinary incontinence reported
Seeing and Sensing	Last ophthalmology visit three years ago; wears prescription tinted sunglasses indoors
	Sensation intact but limited by intention tremor
Shoes and Safety	Wears worn tennis shoes he has had for the last five years; home safety evaluation of daughter's home reveals narrow walkways free of clutter, small bathroom with low rise toilet, and tub with bathroom rugs

the night while ambulating to the bathroom, and the other occurring when his daughter was away from home at work. You complete a COMMSS assessment with the following findings (Table 8.5).

How would you approach this patient to reduce his fall risk?

Feedback: Essential 8 Case Study

- *Fall risk*: Fall risk 4/4—high risk.
  - Number of falls: Greater than three in a year
  - Unsteady gait: Yes
  - Need for a mobility device: Yes, has walker
  - Injury: Yes, vertebral compression fractures

- *Key findings and recommendations*: Dark-tinted sunglasses, screen for DM retinopathy, poor supporting footwear
  - Moderate cognitive impairment—walker placement in view for memory cue for use
  - Parkinson's disease—physical therapy referral
  - Medication adjustment:
    - Stop aspirin to reduce bleeding risk with falls
    - Consider alternative anti-hypertensive to thiazide diuretic (hydrochlorothiazide) with risk of low volume state/electrolyte imbalance increasing fall risk
  - Neurology referral for Parkinson's Disease with tremor management
  - Frequent toileting and use of incontinence briefs
  - Ophthalmology and occupational therapy referrals
  - New supportive, non-skid, rubber-soled shoes
  - DME—bathroom grab bars, shower bench (to lay across tub; patient may sit on and swing his legs over tub rise getting in and out), and toilet riser.
  - Fall prevention education—educate the daughter on providing non-tinted prescription eyeglasses to improve eyesight. Remove throw rugs from the bathroom.

References

1. Office of the US Surgeon General. *The 1964 Report on Smoking and Health*. Washington, DC; 1964.
2. Florence, C. S., & Bergen, G. Medical Costs of Fatal and Nonfatal Falls in Older Adults. *Journal of the American Geriatrics Society*. 2018; 66(4): 693–698.
3. Hoffman, G., & Franco, N. Incidence of and County Variation in Fall Injuries in US Residents Aged 65 Years or Older, 2016–2019. *JAMA Network Open*. 2022; 5(2): 1–4.

CHAPTER 9

Essential 9: Drugs and Ughs

Patient Profile

Presentation: Jesse Donovan, a 73-year-old man with substance abuse history beginning with alcohol and later benzodiazepines. His dependency led to secondary cognitive impairment and alcoholic liver cirrhosis. He is a *high ED utilizer*, mostly for his *primary medical care*, as well as *secondary gain to receive benzodiazepine medications*. Shortly following admission to a high-intensity care program, he again presented back to the ED. This time his presentation was different. He now presented with *extreme fatigue, poor oral intake, and mentation change*. What happened? (See Table 9.1).

Medical management: Complex care comes with complex medicine regimens.

Fundamental 1: *Keep the med list the source of truth.* When other providers, specialists, or hospitals make changes, make sure the med list reflects it. When patients tell you they take the medicine differently than prescribed, update the med list reflecting how it is taken. Yes, this is a labor-intensive process requiring partnership with the medical assistant, RN, and pharmacist,

DOI:10.1201/9781003655084-12

TABLE 9.1   Jesse Donovan, 73-Year-Old Man

Medical History	Medications
Substance abuse history (alcohol, benzodiazepines)	Escitalopram 10 mg daily
Secondary cognitive impairment	Spirinolactone 25 mg daily
Alcoholic liver cirrhosis	Apixaban 5 mg daily
Coronary artery disease (CAD)	Tamsulosin 0.4 mg daily
Heart failure with preserved ejection fraction (HFpEF)	Furosemide 40 mg daily
Chronic obstructive pulmonary disease (COPD)	Albuterol MDI
Atrial fibrillation (AFib)	Fluticasone furoate 100 mcg, umeclidinium 62.5 mch and vilanterol 25 mcg inhalation powder daily
Benign prostatic hyperplasia (BPH)	Isosorbide mononitrate 30 mg daily
Iron deficiency anemia	Clonazepam 0.5 mg bid
Depression with anxiety	Metoprolol 50 mg bid
Gastroesophageal reflux	Omeprazole 20 mg daily
	Tramadol 50 mg q6h prn pain
	Trazodone 50 mg qhs prn sleep

but trust me, there are huge returns in improving outcomes.

Fundamental 2: *Review medications with patients every visit.* Instruct patients in bringing their medications bottles in when assessing medications. *Providers and patients speak different languages when discussing medications (med names versus colors, shapes, or sizes). Looking at the medications together is the translator.* Additionally, patients tend to hang on to discontinued medications. This causes confusion and even inappropriate administration when discontinued medications make their way back into the fold. When evaluating pill bottles, ask them to bring all medications they have in their home. This also affords an opportunity for offering to properly discard unneeded medications.

Polypharmacy is the regular use of five or more medications. It increases the risk of poor outcomes.

This risk increases with age as drug clearance decreases, potentiating drug effects and potential drug interactions. Complex patients have multiple chronic medical conditions, often requiring multiple medicines for control. Attempts at reducing polypharmacy should always be sought accounting for conditions, goals of care, and patient needs. The following description of drug classes help guide decision making for reducing polypharmacy.

Beers Criteria

Several years ago, the American Geriatrics Society published the Beers Criteria of problematic medications in older adults, updated in 2023.[1] It classifies medications into the categories shown in Table 9.2:

Use of medication in higher risk Beers categories should be avoided in complex or elderly patients with strong justification when use is needed.

Antihypertensive Medication

Blood pressure control is important in prevention of stroke, heart attack, and kidney failure. In the frail and elderly, however, physiologic changes associated with aging or chronic disease leave homeostatic compensatory mechanisms diminished. Subtle changes in hydration, for instance, can have devastating effects. We must consider this when setting individualized blood pressure goals and medication titration. Consider also

TABLE 9.2 2023 American Geriatrics Society Beers Criteria

Medications considered as potentially inappropriate

Medications potentially inappropriate in patients with certain diseases or syndromes

Medications to be used with caution

Potentially inappropriate drug–drug interactions

Medications whose dosages should be adjusted based on renal function blood pressure changes with aging. Physiologic age-related weight loss and dietary habits lead to lower baseline blood pressure. *You must consider life expectancy, age, and co-morbidities in setting a goal blood pressure. Allow for permissive hypertension to reduce risk of falls and traumatic injury.*

Remember also Essential 7 (Cognitive Power). Cognitive deficits are common in this population, affecting medication adherence. Blood pressure medications are often titrated up for better control when the real issue is nonadherence or inconsistent adherence due to cognitive decline. Adverse outcomes occurring because of medication adjustments based upon incorrect adherence assumptions are known as the *iatrogenic med assumption.* Our 73-year-old patient example at the beginning of this chapter, Jesse Donovan, is an example of the iatrogenic med assumption. Even though he was prescribed appropriate goal directed therapy for his medical conditions, his cognitive impairment affected medication adherence. Once he enrolled in the high-intensity program and began receiving his medications consistently in blister packs, his adherence increased. Blood pressure medications previously titrated up (assumed subtherapeutic at lower doses) began arriving at his home. A precipitous drop in blood pressure with extreme fatigue, poor PO intake, and decreasing cognition occurred following receiving medications at previously prescribed doses. *Look carefully at blood pressure medications, question adherence, and adjust goals based upon the specifics of the patient.*

Diabetes Medications

In the last 10 years we've seen a revolution in diabetes mellitus management. Technological advances in monitoring and glucose control may well make end-organ destruction (retinopathy, nephropathy, microangiopathy) a vestige of the past, like how disease-modifying antirheumatic drugs (DMARDS) ended the horrific deformities of rheumatoid arthritis. Bioengineering of insulin delivery gave us longer acting insulin with more consistent glucose control. GLP-1 receptor agonists and SGLT inhibitors improve glycemic control and reduce hypoglycemia, with increased cardiac protection. Continuous glucose monitors (CGMs) increase accuracy of monitoring and management with ease of use with an electronic reader or a smartphone. As CGMs become more widely accessible, gone are the days of blaming patients for "not pricking their fingers" for spot checks of glucose readings. However, many complex patients lack access to newer technologies.

Whether on older diabetic management modalities or newer ones, the risk of hypoglycemia still exists in high-risk patients (decreased risk on newer agents). Controversy exists between national endocrine societies on glycemic goals in certain populations including the high risk. HgbA1C is an excellent indicator of longer-term control. Table 9.3 provides a simple guide. (These are not hard and fast rules. Providers need to make clinical decisions at an individual level on each patient. The following recommendations do not replace guidelines or clinical decision-making.)

TABLE 9.3   HgbA1C Goal for Age 65 and Older

Complexity	A1C Goal
Two or fewer stable chronic conditions	Take the patient's age and move the decimal to the left one place so age 70 has goal 7.0, and age 85 has goal 8.5.
Three or more chronic conditions or one uncontrolled	Take the patient's age, add 10, and move the decimal to the left one place (age 82, add 10 to 92, and move decimal one place for goal 9.2).

With goals set, use caution with medication titration. As with blood pressure medications, so too the *iatrogenic med effect* can raise its ugly head with diabetic medications leading to hypoglycemia when diabetic agents are prescribed based upon false adherence assumptions.

Psychoactive Medications

Jesse Donovan traded one dependency (alcohol) for another (benzodiazepines). Both drugs have anxiolytic properties, acting on GABA receptors in the brain. Additionally, both drugs are metabolized by the liver with decreased clearance in liver damage. The effect is the drug, and its effects remain in the system longer, increasing toxicity risk for respiratory depression and death. This happens at lower doses increasing risk of falls, injury, and further decompensation. Medications with sedating properties should be avoided or monitored closely in elderly or medically complex patients. *Review medications with patients every visit.* Adjust medications as appropriate to reduce risk.

Other considerations with psychoactive medications include that many cause orthostatic blood pressure changes. Many have neurologic adverse effects—tardive dyskinesis, Parkinson's like movement disorders, and other extrapyramidal effects. Close monitoring and adjustment are key. Additionally, atypical antipsychotics have a black-box warning of increased risk of death in older adults with dementia-related psychosis because of risk of QT prolongation on EKG leading to increased risk of fatal arrhythmia. Clear and open-ended communication with patients and caregivers with appropriate monitoring with serial EKGs make these medications a viable treatment for those indicated. Prescribers should not shy away from them when they are impactful for their patients.

Pain Medication

Pain management frustrates both providers and patients alike. Unfortunately, science has not unlocked pain relief in the absence of euphoria, setting up for drug abuse. Likewise, narcotics' toxic dose varies between individuals. The narcotic medication class is best at providing acute pain relief; however, its efficacy also varies between individuals. Narcotic medication provides pain relief for some and pain control for others, and still others are only dissociated from the pain—the pain is there but the patient no longer cares (altered perception of pain). Best in mediocrity is nothing to write home about! If that were not complex enough, consider other complexities such as varying pain thresholds, sensitivity to narcotic medication effect or adverse effect, and varying genetic risks to dependency. Currently we do not know who will fall into which group.

Progressive degenerative processes such as osteoarthritis, a ubiquitous inevitability of aging, cause pain syndromes. Advanced age and multiple co-morbidities decrease candidacy of surgical correction. Managing a pain medicine with high pharmacologic tolerance and high abuse and dependency potential is dicey. In the 1990s, pain was adopted as the "fifth vital sign" due to concerns of undertreatment. At the same time, long-acting oral narcotic medications came on the market, touted as breakthrough pain control medications without addictive potential. Unfortunately, both were not true, as abuse, addiction, and overdose deaths rose to epidemic proportions. Consequently, state regulations clamped down with greater oversight and restrictions on prescribing.

Physiology complicates pain management. Acute pain and chronic pain are different processes. Acute pain involves the pain stimuli traveling from the peripheral to the central nervous system mostly via mu receptor synapses. Narcotics work on mu receptors to control pain. After several weeks, pain changes from acute to chronic. Chronic pain occurs when central nervous system pathways involved in pain perception are altered from continuous firing. The peripheral signals may have stopped, but a continuous loop circuit in the brain persists. Hence the brain interprets pain signals from the original peripheral stimulus. Narcotic medications do not work for chronic pain because the perceived pain is not mu receptor peripherally mediated. The neurotransmitters norepinephrine (NE) and serotonin (5HT) are thought to mediate the synaptic responses of the continuous brain loop in chronic pain. Therefore, NE/5HT reuptake inhibitors such as duloxetine have better efficacy in chronic pain.

Chronic pain is best managed without chronic narcotics. Patient education on pain management goals is a must. Level-setting expectations with patients involves understanding pain extinction is not possible. *The goal of pain management is function, not pain elimination.* If the patient can manage daily activities despite pain, goals are met, and further dose adjustment is not indicated. For those who require long-term narcotic medications, best practices include a narcotic contract outlining risks of narcotic medications and conditions of prescribing (at a minimum no early refills, one prescriber and one pharmacy, participating in therapeutic milieu including but not limited to keeping office visits, and no sharing of medications). Additionally, complete a urine drug screening at least annually, and check your state's database of fill history with every new prescription and refill.

Despite greater oversight and formal prescribing guidelines, narcotic dependency in the elderly has risen.[2] Fortunately, an underused, watershed pharmacologic treatment exists. Buprenorphine is life changing for those amenable to its use. States are beginning to remove prescribing restrictions and putting it into the hands of most prescribers. Appropriate dosing is key for avoiding withdrawal and should be done with the assistance of a clinical pharmacist. Cravings subside and patients report it is life enriching, as they are no longer continuously seeking the next narcotic administration.

Medications and the Kidney

Kidney function declines with age. Add to this the fact that the burden of chronic kidney disease due to hypertension and diabetes is of epic proportions. This has two implications. First, we should make every effort at preserving renal function in our complex patients, avoiding medications toxic to the kidney and dosing them appropriately per their renal function. Second, many medications are cleared through the kidneys. Therefore, these medication effects remain in the system and build up, leading to adverse consequences.

Medications that can cause a dehydrated state known as prerenal azotemia must be monitored closely. These include loop diuretics, ACE inhibitors/ARBs, thiazides, neprilysin inhibitors, mineralocorticoid receptor inhibitors, and chemo-therapeutic antimetastatic agents. *Educate patients taking "drying agents" on symptoms of low-volume states with next steps. When starting or titrating these agents, check renal labs in a week, then again in a month.*

Blood Thinners

Everything ages. While age is just a number, we can all think of examples where someone "looks younger than their stated age"—someone whose age says elderly but who is mentally sharp, active, still driving, on little medication, and rarely gets sick. It's the inside that counts. The universal equalizer is microvascular aging. Small vessels in the brain age while outward appearances differ. *Microvascular brain vessels are their stated age.* As such, they are weaker with increased susceptibility to injury. When they are carrying blood with iatrogenic deactivated platelets or altered clotting factors damage has catastrophic consequences.

Macrovascular complications (heart attacks and strokes) have significant morbidity and mortality implications. We must weigh the risk and benefits of anti-platelet and anticoagulation use on individual high-risk patients. This is especially true when they have indications for both medications or dual-antiplatelet management. Give serious consideration of these medications in the frail or high fall risk. Consider alternatives, such as procedures like the left atrial appendage closure, reducing stroke risk, or coming off anticoagulation when bleeding risk is high.

Chapter Summary/Key Takeaways

Medication prescribing is a powerful tool, entrusted to only the most learned and skilled individuals. Medical providers must assess medications frequently in partnership with a clinical pharmacist. Decreasing polypharmacy should always be sought for reducing patient risk.

- Keep the medication list the source of truth. If you are not clear on what the patient is taking, how can you expect them to have a clear understanding?
  - Update with every encounter (in-person, phone, virtual) and transitions of care.
  - Include medications patients taking not prescribed to them, including OTC, vitamins, cannabinoids, and supplements.
  - Remove medications the patient will not take.
  - Instruct patients to bring their medications bottles in when assessing medications so both provider and patient are discussing the same medication at the same time, going

through one by one. *Providers and patients speak different languages when discussing medications (med names versus colors/ shapes/sizes). Looking at the medications together is the translator.*

■ Ancillary staff require training on assessing the complexity of medication compliance. Simple yes-or-no answers to "are you taking this medication" have extremely high reporting errors.

■ Be aware of the iatrogenic med assumption— adverse outcomes stemming from medication adherence assumptions.

■ Use of medication in higher risk Beers categories should be avoided in complex or elderly patients with strong justification when use is needed.

■ Certain medications are high risk in elderly or medically complex patients. Avoidance and reducing polypharmacy, or in special circumstances careful monitoring of the least effective dose, is required. Check for consistency.

■ *Hypertension medications*: Consider life expectancy, age, and co-morbidities in setting a goal blood pressure. Allow for permissive hypertension to reduce risk of falls and traumatic injury.

■ *Diabetes medication:*
  – HgbA1C Goal
    – +65 and less than two controlled chronic conditions: Take their age and move the decimal place left one place (e.g., age 72 goal HgbA1C = 7.2)
    – +65 with at least one chronic condition not controlled or three or more chronic conditions (including DM): Take their age *and add 10* and move

the decimal place left one place (e.g., age 72 goal HgbA1C = 8.2)
- Psychoactive medications
  - Often have cross-tolerance with alcohol and other medications.
  - Medications with sedating properties should be avoided or monitored closely in elderly or medically complex patients.
  - Many have neurologic adverse effects—tardive dyskinesia, orthostatic blood pressure effects, Parkinson's-like movement disorders, and other extrapyramidal effects
  - Atypical antipsychotics have a black-box warning of increased risk of death in older adults with dementia-related psychosis. Clear and open-ended communication with patients and caregivers with appropriate monitoring make these medications a viable treatment for those indicated.
- Narcotic medications
  - Goals are maximizing function over pain control.
  - Chronic pain is not managed best with narcotic medications.
  - In circumstances where chronic narcotic management is needed, titrate to least effective dose and closely monitor with drug testing and entering a shared understanding narcotic contract.
  - With narcotic dependency, consider buprenorphine in consultation with the clinical pharmacist
- Medications affecting the kidneys
  - Educate patients taking "drying agents" on symptoms of low-volume states with next steps.

      – When starting or titrating these agents, check renal function labs in a week, then again in a month.

■ Blood thinners

      – Microvascular brain vessels are their stated age.

      – Weigh risk and benefits of anti-platelet and anticoagulation use on individual high-risk patients.

      – Consider alternatives such as procedures like the left atrial appendage closure, reducing stroke risk, and discontinuing anticoagulation when bleeding risk is high.

Essential 9 Case Study

An 83-year-old female with diabetes mellitus, stage 3b chronic kidney disease, essential hypertension, degenerate disc disease with myelopathy, HFpEF, and depression with anxiety and sleep disturbance presents to primary care to establish care. Her concerns are fatigue, chronic back pain, difficulty sleeping, leg swelling, and vertigo with quick movement upon standing. She walks with the assistance of a 4-pronged cane without history of any recent falls. Her medication list includes:

Amlodipine 5 mg daily
Lisinopril 5/Hydrochlorothiazide 25 mg daily
Glipizide 5 mg/Metformin 500 mg daily
Glargine 25 units nightly
Humalog 5 units tid with meals for blood glucose 200 or greater
Hydrocodone/Acetaminophen 5/325 mg ordered q8h prn but only takes it once or twice a day.
Furosemide 20 mg daily
Paroxetine 10 mg daily
Temazepam 5 mg nightly

Vital Signs: 97.8, 72, 16, 108/65, Pox = 95% RA
MoCA= 24/30
Pertinent Labs: HgbA1C = 7.2%, GFR = 45

How would you approach this patient?

Feedback: Essential 9 Case Study

Advanced age with polypharmacy, reduced renal clearance, vestibular symptoms with fall risk, mild cognitive impairment, and multiple somatic symptoms.

- Review goals:
  - *BP: below target goal.*
  - *DM*- +65 with at least one chronic condition not controlled or three or more chronic conditions (including DM): Take their age *and add 10* and move the decimal place left one place: 83 + 10 = 93, move decimal left 1 place, so target HgbA1C is less than 9.3%.
- Medication list
  - *The patient reports pain and sleep disturbance despite prescribed Hydrocodone/ Acetaminophen and Temazepam. Question adherence, tolerance, or etiology/treatment mismatch, i.e., etiology chronic pain with an acute pain treatment (Norco) prescribed; insomnia secondary to depression (potentially inadequately treated with long-term Paroxetine, an older SSRI) treated with a Temazepam.*
  - *High-risk medications*
    - *Diuretics in the setting of chronic kidney disease (CKD)—loop and thiazide*
    - *Risk of hypoglycemia with HgbA1C below goal*

    – *Paroxetine likely contributes to vestibular symptoms increasing fall risk*
- **Management recommendations**
  - Stop glipizide and metformin for HgbA1C below goal.
  - Stop hydrochlorothiazide given CKD, vestibular symptoms, and propensity for low volume states with co-administration of loop diuretic (furosemide).
  - Stop calcium channel blocker (amlodipine) given concerns over lower extremity edema.
  - Taper off paroxetine and start low-dose mirtazapine at night for sleep and depression, which will likely improve perception of pain control.
  - Follow-up in 1 week to 1 month for BP check, repeat renal function testing, and review of blood glucose logs.

Ughs

Patient care challenges can make you go, "Ugh." Over the years I've developed words of wisdom, pearls if you will, affectionately called Ughs for their initial reaction namesake. Some nest nicely with the 9 Essentials. Others do not necessarily fit neatly into any one essential (and some bear repeating). Because they are powerful and high-yield, I wanted to make sure they were included. Enjoy reading through this section. I believe you will find them as useful as I do.

☺ Patient Assessment Is Better Done *in Vivo* than *in Vitro*

I am honored and privileged caring for patients in their home. Patients trust their providers on the most intimate aspects of their lives. This multiplies exponentially when they allow you into their home lives. I'll never forget one of my first home visits with a 66-year-old veteran, Ms. Bradshaw. She lived alone in her one-bedroom apartment. Her body was aged beyond her numeric years. Unfortunately, she now required supplemental oxygen secondary to smoking-induced chronic obstructive pulmonary disease (COPD). Ms. Bradshaw had poor functional exercise capacity, severely limiting her activity, with frequent exacerbations. She had mild cognitive dysfunction per screening tests. Additionally, she was prescribed continuous positive airway pressure (CPAP) for obstructive sleep apnea (OSA).

I asked Ms. Bradshaw about her compliance with CPAP. The benefits of use of continuous airway positive pressure for her include improved lung compliance, functional ability, and reduced COPD exacerbations. Ms. Bradshaw reported she did not use her CPAP because she could not tolerate the pressures at night (a common finding among OSA patients). At this point I would normally give my spiel on benefits of CPAP, recommendations for refitting, use of CPAP while awake for becoming accustomed to it, use of the low pressure setting while falling asleep, and finally that any use is better than no use—benefits are seen with a couple hours use at night versus no use. But something happened, forever changing my approach with OSA patients.

Ms. Bradshaw asked that I observe her use of CPAP. The nurse and I walked with Ms. Bradshaw into her bedroom. Ms. Bradshaw pulled out her CPAP mask and began putting it on. It was apparent that she lacked the dexterity for adjusting the multiple straps for securing a tight fit. Additionally, her problem-solving ability, including concentration for securing a tight fit, was compromised due to her cognitive dysfunction. Because she also required supplemental oxygen, it required disconnecting from her nasal cannula and reconnecting it to the CPAP hose connector. I assisted, and even I had some difficulty with this technical task. I can only imagine how difficult this must be on a frail, elderly individual with mild cognitive impairment! The problem is not inability tolerating

CPAP (as often reported); the problem is difficulty doing the steps required for compliance. You get a different perspective when observing patients in their environment versus an office environment.

Reducing Utilization from CHF/COPD

☹ The Frequent Exacerbator

It takes two to Tango: chronic disease management requires continual assessment by provider *and* patient.

Despite a large base of knowledge, many patients and families have little understanding of self-management.[3] Many ED visits are preventable if patients and caregivers recognize early signs of exacerbations, how to reverse them, and how to receive help when they are not improving. One of the highest yield interventions is spending time educating patients that chronic disease is not curable but manageable. It is going to take effort on their part, evaluating daily, but the returns are huge: fewer days in the hospital, more time at home with loved ones, more days feeling better, and improved overall quality of life (including increased activity and exercise tolerance). There are several materials to help you, including local health systems' "red, yellow, and green stoplight tools" with signs, symptoms, and directions for assistance and management.

In COPD or congestive heart failure (CHF), evaluate these conditions every office visit. Changes can be subtle, even for the most experienced providers. Objective data collection is needed, i.e., validated COPD symptoms, assessment tools, weight logs, etc.

☹ Illness Doesn't Work at the Bank

Patients must have direct access to a provider when there is an exacerbation. Exacerbations occur outside of Monday–Friday, 8–5. A large part of unnecessary ED utilization occurs due to poor access to care.

Primary care offices are booked during the day and utilize nursing call centers after hours. Unfortunately, this is often done without physician intervention. The more direct care, the better. Many providers give out their personal cell phone numbers. I am not necessarily advocating this approach, but older or cognitively impaired chronically ill patients often struggle navigating a phone tree. Patients must trust that when they're in trouble, they can get help. Don't be surprised when first starting a high-risk program with direct provider access after-hours if patients still utilize the ED. People often neglect other options and go right to ED. Often these are ingrained behaviors—how they are used to receiving urgent care. Start developing trust that you can safely help them outside of an ED visit after hours.

☹ Show Your Work on the Refrigerator

Just like a parent placing a child's schoolwork on the refrigerator, have patients do the same with their chronic disease patient assessment tools (stoplight tools, etc.). It's a memory aid for daily assessment.

COPD self-management includes daily monitoring of cough, shortness of breath/activity level, and rescue medication use.

- Monitor for change in cough type (productive, nonproductive, etc.) and frequency.
- Change in sputum—color, consistency, or amount.
- Change in shortness of breath symptoms: Previously short of breath with moderate activity and now with minimal activity?
- Use of rescue medication: Are you using rescue medication more frequently?

For severe exacerbations—unable to clear secretions, shortness of breath at rest, hypoxia/cyanosis, no response to rescue medication—go to the ED.

☺ Provider Assessment of COPD

1. Validated COPD symptom assessment tool every visit to assess for change.
2. Assess rescue medication use—technique and frequency.
3. Lung auscultation examination.

CHF self-management includes *daily* monitoring of weight log, shortness of breath/activity, sodium/fluid intake, and peripheral edema. Notify provider for:

- Weight increase of 2 lbs. or more in 24 hours. Highly consider standing additional prn diuretic dosing.
- Edema moving from feet or ankles up lower extremities or even to abdomen.
- Change in shortness of breath symptoms: Were they previously short of breath with moderate activity and now with minimal activity?

For severe CHF exacerbations—anasarca, shortness of breath at rest, hypoxia/cyanosis, anuria—go to the ED.

☺ Provider Assessment of CHF Includes Review of *Daily* Weight Log, Physical Exam, and BNP Trend

☺ *SABA Right Along*
Frequent short-acting beta agonists (SABAs) reduce symptom severity.

- Mild to moderate COPD exacerbations: Use rescue medication q4-6h × 24 hours. Notify the access line for worsening symptoms or no improvement after 24 hours.
- Nebulized Albuterol before bed and first thing in the morning wards off evil spirits (and reduces exacerbations too)!

- Use a nebulizer when at home and save inhalers for when away from home or otherwise without access to the nebulizer. Nebulized medication delivery is superior to metered delivery devices.

Let's Check Your Technique

The pharmaceutical industry created a plethora of inhaler delivery devices including metered dose inhalers, dry powder inhalers, and soft mist inhalers. Each type requires a certain administration technique and can be challenging to a high-risk patient with cognitive deficits, low vision/dexterity, and deconditioning. Check, correct, and teach proper technique. Switch medication/inhaler types if it becomes apparent a patient cannot manage a certain inhaler type.

I Heart Kidneys

To avoid cardio-renal syndrome:

1. Only prescribe diuretics for peripheral edema for the following reasons:
   a. Evidence of co-morbid pulmonary edema
   b. Associated extremity pain
   c. Inability to put on shoes or edema makes it difficult to safely ambulate.
2. Absence of symptoms in item 1—treat peripheral edema with lower extremity elevation, compression socks, and Na/fluid restriction.

COPD Non-Responder: Think BNP!

Congestive heart failure can be a masquerader. Symptomatic pulmonary edema can occur without rales/crackles on auscultation or curly B lines on x-ray. Mild interstitial edema has a huge effect on lungs already inflamed and damaged by COPD. A little diuresis or keeping a severe COPD patient a little on the dry side often decreases breathlessness and reduces trips to the hospital.

☹ The Chicken or the Egg?

Which came first, dyspnea or panic? If you've ever gone without oxygen for more than a few seconds, panic sets in. However, a sympathetic fight or flight response to the stress in this scenario is counterproductive because it creates an oxygen supply/demand mismatch. You need more oxygen for flight or flight when less is available. But what if anxiety set in first? Sympathetic response increases respiratory rate and oxygen need, but with COPD, it cannot deliver. Now we're back to the first scenario where hypoxia drives panic. It's a vicious cycle and sometimes an anxiolytic like alprazolam at low doses reduces anxiety, slows respiratory rate, and increases time for gas exchange decreasing air-hunger.

☹ Anyone Got a Used Cola Bottle?

The easiest method for monitoring daily 2 L fluid restriction: Fill an empty 2 L bottle with water and pour out an equal part of water for every liquid drank. When the 2 L bottle is empty, no more fluid for the day. It's a visual for the patient on how much fluid is left for the day and beats the heck out of measuring and adding amounts! And if it's on the rocks, don't forget to count the ice cubes!

☹ Na's Hide and Seek

Food with hidden salt: Bread, sandwiches, cold cut meats, canned foods including soups and vegetables, pizza, tacos, and pretty much anything eating out.

☹ Go for the GOLD

Follow Global Initiative for Chronic Obstructive Lung Disease (GOLD) guidelines for medication prescribing. Aggressively step up therapy appropriately. GOLD guidelines are as follows[5]:

■ Long-acting muscarinic antagonists (LAMAs) are preferred over inhaled corticosteroids in COPD.

☺ Only water increases weight 2 or more pounds in 24 hours.

Psychosocial and Behavioral
☹ Home Environment: What's Going on at Home?

The home environment is very telling. Assess:

- Medications: locations, container types
- Animals: pets and otherwise
- Working utilities
- Clutter/fall risks
- Who's home
- Food

☺ Got Support?

When we get stuck, often there is a friend or family member who can help. Engaging social support early increases the odds of success. A great question for patients is: "If you needed assistance, who would you call?"

☹ Patient Reluctance for Behavioral Health Services

- Evaluate sleep, prescribe mirtazapine

Patients are more accepting of medications for indication of sleep rather than a psychiatric diagnosis. They are much more accepting of taking mirtazapine for sleep than taking it for mood stabilization.

☺ A Multi-Somatic Complainer Has Depression Until Proven Otherwise

☺ *You Don't Have to Get Snippy: The Angry Patient*

- Anger shows frustration with navigating the system and/or acceptance of condition—go to empathy techniques.

- For personality disorders: set clear boundaries and maintain them.

☹ For the Obstinate Patient with Dementia, It's About Control—Give It to Them!

We all want control of our lives. As we age and become more dependent on others, we naturally begin losing some control. This causes conflict. Give patients control with choices that don't really matter in the scheme of things but give the patient control of the choice, i.e., what to wear, what to eat, where to go, etc.

☹ The Sky Can Be Many Colors Other Than Blue

Arguing with a dementia patient is futile. Unless it's a matter of safety (don't touch the hot stove), don't argue about who did what, when things occurred, or who you are. If they say the sky's not blue, agree with them that it's red, green, or polka-dot.

☹ A Poor Memory Has Its Advantages

Distraction works well in short-term memory deficits. A patient with dementia will often not remember to go back to the unwanted activity. Distraction techniques include looking at old photo albums, listening to music, or turning on a television program.

☹ Dementia Involves Good Days and Bad Days

In early dementia there are more good days than bad. In late dementia there are more bad days than good. It's a mix in moderate dementia.

Cognition and functional status wax and wane in dementia, especially in moderate to late stages. When altered mentation occurs in the setting of positive urinary culture, in the absence of urinary signs and symptoms, it is colonization, rather than infection, requiring no further treatment. Educate families on risks of inappropriate antibiotic use including resistance and pathogenic overgrowth.

☹ Weakness: If Not for the Weak ...

Stroke deficits recur with weakness or illness. Following rehabilitation, stroke deficits can diminish or resolve as the patient learns compensatory mechanisms. However, when an acute illness sets in, the patient's compensatory mechanisms decrease and the deficit recurs. Patients and families become concerned for a stroke recurrence. Patient education on this phenomenon helps reassure and set expectations, reducing unnecessary trips to the ED.

☹ Pain Management: What a Pain!

The chronic pain management patient is challenging. For patients presenting with the following ailments, look for narcotic medication etiology.

- AMS
- Constipation
- Fall(s)
- Diarrhea—Chronic narcotic medication present with diarrhea (acute or chronic) as patients overuse, run out of medications, and withdraw.

☹ Back Pain or Decreased Urinary Stream in a Male Patient: Assess for Constipation

Constipation occurs when retained stool in the colon puts pressure on the prostatic urethra, decreasing its stream. Colon distension can also refer pain to the low back.

Medication Management
☺ Containers over Bottles

With multiple medications, especially with multiple administrations a day, pill containers are preferred over taking pills from the bottles. The organization is systematic. In cases where a family member may need to step in and assist in medication administration, it is more streamlined. The organization is a visual of doses needed versus doses taken (Did I take my morning meds? If I check a bottle full of pills, there is no way to know unless you do pill counts, but if you look at the container you can see if they are there or already taken.)

☹ We're Not Speaking the Same Language

Remember providers and patients speak different medication languages; what to some is metoprolol to another is the white pill.

☹ Avoid Thiazides in Older or Complex Patients

Dehydration, acute kidney injury, hypokalemia, and gout flares are more prominent adverse effects in this population.

☺ Recurrent UTI in Diabetes: Ensure Glycemic Control

Hyperglycemia decreases immune response with increased infections. Hyperglycemia is a neurotoxin including micturition nerves leading to neurogenic bladder with urinary retention, urine pooling, and infection.

☺ Goals of Care

If you're finding yourself pleading with a patient to go to the ED or hospital, ask yourself if a goals-of-care discussion is more appropriate.

9 Essentials Case Study—Conclusion

With Marie's expression of emotion, the nurse manager Katie's demeanor changed instantly. Katie's Cardinal Truth showed, an overwhelming sense of empathy for Marie came over Katie. "Marie, I can only imagine how difficult this is for you. We've known each other awhile, I remember when you, your dad, and family were here with your mother. I remember how much your dad struggled between keeping your mom comfortable and respecting her religious beliefs of preserving life. Did he ever talk about what he wanted in a similar situation?"

"Oh yes, it tore him up seeing my mother like that. He said he never wanted to suffer like that. He respected mom's church beliefs, but he also told us he didn't believe God wanted people suffering. He said, 'Don't let this happen to me. When my time comes, don't keep me lingering.' It's so hard though, he's, my dad. I know he's hard to manage but I'm not sure if he's suffering."

"Thank you for sharing, Marie, I know that must have been difficult." Katie said. "Your dad really empathized with your mother, putting himself in her shoes, courageously communicating he would not want the same. Marie, have you given any thought to if you were in your dad's position? What would you want?"

Marie's facial expression shifted. You could see she was deep in thought. "I wouldn't want any of this. Yes, he is suffering, I see that now."

"Marie, could we talk about other options where the goal is comfort, quality over quantity of life?"

References

1. 2023 American Geriatrics Society Beers Criteria Update Expert Panel. American Geriatrics Society 2023 Updated AGS Beers Criteria for Potentially

Inappropriate Medication Use in Older Adults. *Journal of the American Geriatrics Society.* 2023; 71(7): 2052–2081.

2. Huhn, A. S., Strain, E. C., Tompkins, D. A., et al. A Hidden Aspect of the U.S. Opioid Crisis: Rise in First-Time Treatment Admissions for Older Adults with Opioid Use Disorder. *Drug Alcohol Dependence.* 2018; 193: 142–147.

3. Laura, M., Mackey, C. D., Doody, C., Werner, E. L., et al. Self-Management Skills in Chronic Disease Management: What Role Does Health Literacy Have? *Medical Decision Making.* 2016; 36(6): 741–759.

4. American Thoracic Society. *How Is Your COPD? Take the COPD Assessment Test (CAT).* June 25, 2023. https://www.researchgate.net/figure/Evaluative-questions-from-the-COPD-Assessment-Test-CAT-COPD-Assessment-Test-and-the_fig1_244482870

5. Agusti, A., Celli, B. R., Criner, G. J., et al. Global Initiative for Chronic Obstructive Lung Disease 2023 Report: GOLD Executive Summary. *American Journal of Respiratory and Critical Care Medicine.* 2023; 207(7): 813–819.

Epilogue/Conclusion

The Rodriguez family story illustrates successfully managing a challenging, complex patient through the 9 Essentials of Quality Care. As is commonly seen, the care team experienced learned helplessness due to the carry burden of the weight of ensuring their patient's safety. They began believing a resolute fallacy: Marie, the patient's daughter, was incapable of change. This culminated in intellectual paralysis, essentially giving up and recommending discharge of services. Marie's reaction awakened the cardinal truth (deep down, every health care provider wants to help patients) in Katie, the RN manager, who then approached differently.

An epiphany occurred. There is hope in this seemingly impossible case. No one is beyond help (Essential 1). When there is no improvement, you have not reached the barrier. In this case, the barrier is confliction of Essential 2 (the right care, in the right place, at the right time). Mr. Rodriguez's aggressive care model did not match his needs. In fact, repeated hospitalizations furthered his decline. His metaphorical medevac helicopter ride (risks of higher-level care) risk is too high. The right care is palliative.

The care team got stuck with "we know best"—a take-it-or-leave-it recommendation. We've seen this

DOI:10.1201/9781003655084-13

before; we are the experts; we know what's best! Marie's emotional response uncovered what mattered most for the Rodriguez family—comfort with dignity, remaining out of the nursing home. To meet 'em where they are and bring them along (Essential 6), Katie had to check her ego at the door (Essential 3). She let go of her self-righteous approach and began demonstrating her cardinal truth through body language and empathetic statements (Essential 5: I Care). This allowed movement, aligning patient and family desires with appropriate goals of care.

Opportunities were missed in care team collaboration. Improved team dynamics would likely facilitate other perspectives, uncovering barriers to care (Essential 4: You Cannot Dot It Alone). Darla-Kay's observed worsening undesirable behaviors with Marie's interactions with Mr. Rodriguez. There was a missed opportunity for team recognition for dementia education (allow for perceptions of patient control—give choices, be nonconfrontational, etc.) (Essential 7: Cognitive Power). Other opportunities for Mr. Rodriguez involve recurrent falls (Essential 8: Gotta Move) and medications (Essential 9: Drugs and Ughs) especially as they relate to disruptive behaviors.

Managing complex patients, more prevalent in health care, is challenging. Without a roadmap, well-intended health care professionals fall into common pitfalls. For success, you need to *change thinking*—realize you can affect change, let go of your pride, level-set with your interdisciplinary team and patients with empathy, compassion, and shared goals. Systematically assess cognition, mobility, and medication management with wisdom and experience. Be the health care professional at the right place and time, helping patients reach their health care goals.

Index

Pages in *italics* refer to figures and pages in **bold** refer to tables.

P

partnership with patient, 99, 103–104
patient discharge/dismissal, 88
Patient Health Questionnaire-9
(PHQ-9), 7
permissive hypertension, 135, 142
personal construct theory (PCT), 36, **39**
Peterson, Christopher, 8
physical/occupational therapy, 27, **52**,
75, 122, **125**, **129**, 131
polypharmacy, 133–134, 141–142, 145
preventative care, 23, 30, 122
Program for the All-Inclusive Care of
the Elderly (PACE), 21, 38, 60
pseudodementia, 114, 116

R

rapport, 38, 68, 76–77, 82–83
building in relationships, 53, 57,
91–92
in case studies, 40, 87–88, **89–90**, 102
culturally aware, 84–85
rehabilitation, 22, 27, 52, 123,
128, 155; *see also* subacute
rehabilitation
rehabilitation therapist, 41
relative value units (RVUs), 25
resolute fallacy, 12–15, 17, 54, 61, 87,
158

S

Salovey, Peter, 38
Seligman, Martin, 8, 57–59
short-acting beta agonists (SABAs), 150

social determinants of health
(SDOH), 57, 104
social support, 53, 91, **94**, **124**, 126,
153
in case studies, 13, 64, 76; *see also*
language interpreters
subacute rehabilitation (SAR), 15–16,
27, 123

T

teams, 48, 76, 84, 100, 103
managing and building,
51–60, 62
leadership of, 48–51, 60, 62–63,
65–69

U

urgent care, 26, 149
utilization
of emergency departments (EDs), 3,
5, 9–10, 12, 57, 148
of hospitals, 15, 22, 26, 53
metrics of, 3, 36
reducing, 6, 60, 63

V

value, 55, 57–58, 62, 101
value-based care, 21–26, 29–30, 65
Veterans Equitable Resource Allocation
(VERA), 22
Veterans Health Administration (VHA),
22
vulnerability, 59, 63, 66, 68–69

For Product Safety Concerns and Information please contact our EU
representative GPSR@taylorandfrancis.com
Taylor & Francis Verlag GmbH, Kaufingerstraße 24, 80331 München, Germany

www.ingramcontent.com/pod-product-compliance
Lightning Source LLC
Chambersburg PA
CBHW061313220326
41599CB00026B/4853

* 9 7 8 1 0 4 1 1 0 4 5 0 6 *